ADDITIVE ALERT

YOUR GUIDE TO SAFER SHOPPING

The essential information about
what's *really* in the food you eat,
which additives to avoid and why

JULIE EADY

FULLY REVISED THIRD EDITION

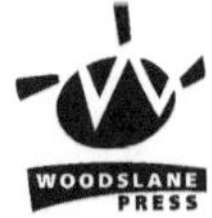

Woodslane Press Pty Ltd
10 Apollo Street
Warriewood, NSW 2102
Email: info@woodslane.com.au
Tel: 02 8445 2300 Website: www.woodslanepress.com.au

First edition published in Australia in 2004 by Additive Alert Pty Ltd.
Second edition published in 2006 by Additive Alert Pty Ltd, revised 2008 and 2010.
Re-issued second edition published in Australia in 2016 by Woodslane Press Pty Ltd.
This fully revised and updated third edition published by Woodslane Press Pty Ltd
in September 2017.
Reprinted 2018.
Now printed in Australia via POD

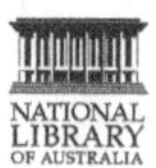
A catalogue record for this
book is available from the
National Library of Australia

Cover design by Jenny Cowan

Julie Eady was a full time Mum to three young children, a devoted wife, friend and consumer advocate. On September 26th 2017, she died suddenly due to complications of a blood infection. She was 50 years old. Julie developed her interest in food additives and their effects on health after the birth of her first child in 1999. With a family history of allergies and asthma, she began her research into dietary links to such illnesses, in an effort to improve her children's chances of avoiding these conditions.

What began as a personal project to identify better food choices for her family, led onto a much bigger project as she discovered the truth about the serious health concerns associated with many additives used in Australian foods.

Julie's vision for Additive Alert is to promote better consumer awareness of food additives and their effects on health, and to advocate for better labelling of Australian foods. In March 2007 Julie was awarded the Western Australian Consumer Protection Award, in recognition of her work as a consumer advocate and the benefits her work with Additive Alert has brought to the community.

Julie's mission was to spread her message and raise awareness about the effects of food additives through her book and a busy public speaking schedule, which she maintained for many years. From 2004 she delivered her popular Additive Alert presentations at hundreds of schools, community groups and corporate events, and became a regular guest on popular television and radio shows. Her information and advice always generated a huge response from listeners wanting to know more about how additives can affect their health.

Julie's home was in the Perth beachside suburb of Mullaloo where she lived with her husband Stuart and children Jaslyn, Mitchell and Jonothan. She enjoyed living a healthy life by the beach. Her favourite places to holiday were Rottnest Island, Kingscliff in northern NSW and Broome and the Kimberley, where she loved to escape the winter chills as often as possible. Julie lived an outstanding life. She achieved so much more than she ever envisaged and was one of the fortunate few to have a life of true happiness and love.

Disclaimer

This book has been compiled from the author's own research and personal experiences. The content is not intended to constitute scientific or medical advice or to include all information about all additives used in food. Every effort has been made to ensure that the information contained in this book is accurate and current at the time of publication.

Numerous existing public references were consulted and cross-referenced in preparing this book and in determining the health risks attributed to certain additives. The author does not guarantee the accuracy of the information obtained from the sources or cited references and disclaims liability for the accuracy of that information. The author also does not endorse, recommend or promote any product over another.

The author acknowledges that product content may change from time to time and welcomes product updates for any products cited in this book so that any omissions, errors or additive changes can be corrected in future editions.

Additive Alert: Your Guide to Safer Shopping is intended to enable readers to form their own judgments about which products best suit their individual needs. The author disclaims liability for any use, misuse or misunderstanding of any information contained herein, or for any loss, damage or injury (be it health, financial or otherwise) for any individual or group acting upon or relying on information contained in or inferred from this work.

A qualified health practitioner should always be consulted about individuals' health requirements and any significant dietary changes.

Acknowledgements

The idea for this work first glimmered in 2002, and it then took two and a half years to finish in between looking after our daughter Jaslyn and welcoming Mitchell into our family.

My special thanks therefore go to my husband Stuart and wonderful children Jaslyn, Mitchell and Jonothan, for their love and understanding for my "time off" in the office and countless hours in supermarkets surveying product ingredients.

My thanks also to the rest of my family – Jocelyn, Mark, Helen and Ross - for their unwavering encouragement and support, their positive contributions and suggestions and mostly for their babysitting. A special thanks also to Dr Peter Dingle for being so generous with his time and expertise. His enthusiasm and encouragement gave me the inspiration to believe that small steps taken by ordinary people can make a big difference, and the courage to ensure that this book was finished.

Finally, I owe a huge thank you to the thousands of people who have read Additive Alert already and who have supported our campaigns for safer products for Australian consumers. Together we have influenced our regulators, politicians and the food industry. I have seen a huge improvement in our product choices since 2004, but we still have a long way to go. To all of you who have supprted our campaigns, come along to talks, shared the information with friends and families or just quietly changed your shopping habits to support safe additive products, you have all helped to make a very big difference.

I wrote this book originally in the hope that it would make a difference in some small way to the health and wellbeing of others. 13 years later, I know for sure that this has happened, thanks to the many emails and letters I have received confirming the huge role that additives can have on health, especially in children. I am disappointed that our food regulator still refuses to put consumer safety before manufacturers' interests, but I am inspired by our combined power as consumers to effect change. I am grateful every day for my 3 healthy children. I hope that Additive Alert continues to help other families and that we will continue to see less and less of the nasty additives in our foods.

Foreword

Have you ever wondered why we have increasing rates of childhood illness despite the increasing amounts of money we put into our health system? Do you wonder why rates of cancer, ADHD, depression, suicide and even cardiovascular disease continue to rise in children? The reason is clear. We do not have a system that creates health. We have a pharmaceutical-based health system that treats the symptoms and not the disease.

In Australia each month **60000** prescriptions for antidepressants are written out for people under **20** years of age, and this is on the increase.

If we had a health system, it would be targeting our poor Diets, our contaminated Environment, our negative Attitude and our stressed Lifestyle. Something I call the DEAL, rather than prescribing medications that have serious side effects and, at best, only short-term benefits.

If you are interested in good health, where do you start? I suggest you look at what you put in your mouth, particularly the food additives.

Many food additives are cosmetic ingredients used for the sole purpose of fooling the consumer. Did you know that most have no benefit and many have serious adverse effects? Research over the past 40 years has linked many of the artificial food colours derived from petrol with ADHD and certain allergic reactions. The chemicals that form the preservatives put into processed meats definitely cause cancer and are directly linked with childhood leukaemia. This scares me because I see many children eating lots of processed meats in the form of luncheon meats, sausages, frankfurts and party sausages.

On top of this, the foods containing most of these additives are targeted to the most vulnerable group in our population, our children. Children are much more vulnerable because their bodies are growing and laying down their foundation for health for the rest of their lives. Numerous studies have shown children react more severely to many of these toxic food additives than adults.

Yet, every year, food manufacturers target advertising at youth, to fool them into believing that these over-processed foods with lots of additives and no nutrition are going to bring some benefit - either social, psychological, emotional or physical. Have you ever wondered why you never see a really obese group of kids with ADHD and depression on a soft drink or lolly advertisement?

You need to know the hard facts about food additives and that they are a significant contributing factor to our kids' poor health.

My utopia in the future will not put our kids' health at risk. Future governments will put our health first and economics second. Governments will not allow substances to be added to foods unless they benefit our kids and add some nutrition, and industry will substitute beneficial additives and go back to putting real food in our food.

But until such a utopia arrives, you need to learn as much as you can about food additives and change what you can in your own lives. Do this by reading this book.

Dr Peter Dingle
Environmental and Nutritional Toxicologist
School of Environmental Science
Murdoch University
www.drdingle.com

Author of
The DEAL for Happier, Healthier, Smarter Kids: A Twenty First Century Guide for Parents

Contents

Disclaimer iv

Acknowledgements v

Foreword vi

Introduction xi

Chapter 1: About this book 1
   1.1   Introduction 1
   1.2   What this book tells you and what it doesn't 3

Chapter 2: Food additives: what and why? 5
   2.1   Introduction 5
   2.2   The functions of food additives 6
   2.3   Additive numbers 8
   2.4   Additives explosion 9

Chapter 3: Additives and health concerns 11
   3.1   A picture of health 11
   3.2   So what's going on? 17
   3.3   Could it be the food? 19
   3.4   Food allergies and food intolerance 20

Chapter 4: Your health, your choice 25

Chapter 5: Regulation in Australia 29

Chapter 6: Testing and approval of additives 33
   6.1   The current system 33
   6.2   So what's the problem? 34

Chapter 7: Understanding labels 39
   7.1   Introduction 39
   7.2   Numbers or names? 40
   7.3   The 5% loophole 40
   7.4   No warnings 41

Chapter 8: Labelling licence: what you need to know 43

    8.1   Reading ingredient labels 43

    8.2   Hidden additives 44

    8.3   No-MSG claims 45

    8.4   Natural colour 45

    8.5   Flavours 46

    8.6   Organic claims 47

    8.7   No artificial preservatives 48

    8.8   Advertising by omission 48

    8.9   Customer enquiry services 48

Chapter 9: The ones to watch out for 51

    9.1   MSG and flavour enhancers 51

    9.2   Avoiding MSG isn't as easy as it should be 55

    9.3   Ways to disguise MSG in foods 56

    9.4   Aspartame and artificial sweeteners 58

    9.5   Other artificial sweeteners 61

    9.6   Nitrates and nitrites 64

    9.7   Artificial colours 67

    9.8   Preservatives 72

    9.9   Sulphites (220–228) 73

    9.10   Propionates (280–283) 76

    9.11   Benzoates (210–213) 78

    9.12   Dried fruit and fresh fruit 80

    9.13   Antioxidants 82

    9.14   Propyl, octyl and dodecyl-gallate (310–312) 83

    9.15   Tert-butylhydroquinone or TBHQ (319) 83

    9.16   Butylated hydroxyanisole or BHA (320) 83

    9.17   Butylated hydroxytoluene or BHT (321) 84

    9.18   Avoiding the nasty antioxidants – can it be done? .. 84

Chapter 10: So what's left? 85

    10.1   Decision time 85

    10.2   Changing the habits of a lifetime 86

Chapter 11: Healthier low-additive eating guidelines 89
    11.1   Introduction 89
    11.2   Increase your fruit and vegetable consumption 90
    11.3   Go organic if you can 91
    11.4   Drink more water 92
    11.5   Eliminate fizzy drinks and cordials 92
    11.6   Choose no-additive juices 93
    11.7   Bread 94
    11.8   Butter, margarine and spreads 96
    11.9   Low fat and lite products 99
    11.10 Salt 100
    11.11 Sugar 101
    11.12 Whole grains 103
    11.13 Cooking sauces and flavour bases 105
    11.14 Two-minute noodles and pasta snacks 106
    11.15 Avoid processed meats 107
    11.16 Party food 108
    11.17 Foods for young children 111
    11.18 Smarter rewards 113
    11.19 Reset your bliss point 115

Chapter 12: Get to it: take control of your kitchen 117
    12.1   Introduction 117
    12.2   Additive consumption comparison 120

Chapter 13: Taking it further by forcing change 127

Appendix 1: Additives to avoid 131

Appendix 2: Consumer information lines 135

Appendix 3: Useful contacts 136

Appendix 4: Additive effects 140

Appendix 5: Food Additives Alphabetical Listing 158

References 170

Introduction

Most people want to be healthy and avoid disease and illness. Most parents, in particular, want their children to be healthy and safe and wouldn't dream of intentionally feeding or exposing them to dangerous chemicals or toxins. Unfortunately, most of us have little idea about the chemicals and toxins we're exposed to every day in our environment, and worse, through the food we eat.

The following examples may shock you, but — incredibly — they are real.

- Many brands of peanut butter in Australia contain a particularly nasty chemical known as butylated hydroxyanisole (BHA). This chemical is known to cause stomach cancer in rats and mice and is strongly thought to be a human carcinogen also. Usually there's no mention of this additive on the label due to a loophole in the labelling laws in this country. Other equally effective, non-toxic additives exist that can do the same job, but BHA is cheaper and so is more widely used.

- Ice cream cones, you'd think, wouldn't contain many additives, and, if they did, surely they would be guaranteed to be safe? Think again. Most popular brands contain at least three artificial colours that are linked to hyperactivity and behavioural problems in children, are known animal carcinogens, and are also proven mutagens (agents that cause damage to DNA). In addition, many of these products also contain the antioxidant BHA, mentioned above.

- Baby food is protected under legislation from the addition of many of the more toxic food additives. Even so, throughout the research for this book, examples were found of well known baby foods that contained additives which are known animal carcinogens and mutagens, as well as colours and preservatives which have been shown to promote hyperactivity in children and which are also proven asthma triggers.

There are many more disturbing examples of toxic chemicals in the food we eat everyday, some of which I will share with you throughout this book. These "additives" aren't food–they are toxic chemicals–and they have no place in our diet.

Thankfully, many food additives are harmless and may be beneficial, but there are numerous food additives still in use today that are known to be dangerous and which, given the choice, most of us would choose not to consume or feed to our families.

You are probably thinking, "How can this be true? Surely it is illegal in Australia to put toxic chemicals in the food we buy?" Unfortunately, it isn't. Of the 300 or so permitted food additives in Australia, at least 30 are regarded internationally as suspected carcinogens. This means that these additives have been shown definitely to cause carcinogenic effects in animal studies, and yet they are still permitted in "safe doses" in our foods. Many others have previously been banned or phased out of use in other countries because of their known adverse effects, and yet Australia lags behind and continues to permit their usage in a huge array of our everyday foods such as fruit juice, yoghurts, cereals, museli bars, biscuits and more.

The reason for this appalling double standard is simply that the Australian approach to regulation of food chemicals is not as rigorous or *precautionary* as that applied in many other countries. In some countries, a food additive will be banned outright if it is seen to cause any cancerous effects, at any level, in any animal studies.

Astoundingly though, in Australia this *precautionary principle* is not applied universally when evaluating the safety of food additives. This is why so many of our food and drinks products still quite legally contain numerous food additives which have been shown to cause carcinogenic, mutagenic and teratogenic (agents that cause birth defects) effects in animals studies. More about this and the short comings of our regulation of food additives in Australia can be found in *Chapter 6: Testing and approval of additives.*

Despite all this, however there is some very good news to share. There is an abundance of great low additive, healthier choices available in our supermarkets today. We don't have to accept the substandard products containing unsafe or questionable additives. Even with the increasing prevalence of food additives in our food, across the board there are smart food choices that the informed consumer can make.

We can greatly reduce our daily intake of unnecessary, and often unsafe, food chemicals and toxins simply by choosing products that don't contain these dangerous substances. Thankfully, there are still products with little or no "nasty" additives in them, and these are the products we should be supporting.

The food-manufacturing industry is big business. There is a vast amount of energy and money invested by the food industry into packaging goods to be appealing to customers. In some cases, downright misleading and false statements are made to reassure consumers about the safety of products. For example, undesirable ingredients are listed using long and complex chemical names and numbers, or are simply not declared at all.

The reality is, that although most people would like to be better informed about the food they eat and what is in it, most of us can't find the time to read and understand food labels. The people who most often do are the people who have to — usually those with a health problem or those with a child or family member with an illness or health concern. Most of us are simply too busy to take on this task and we assume and hope that the food we buy must be safe. Unfortunately this isn't always the case, even in Australia.

But relax, keep reading and don't panic!

You don't have to become a label-reading expert or a dedicated home scientist to decipher all the chemical names, numbers and symbols, to eliminate many of these suspect chemicals from your family's diet.

Additive Alert: Your Guide to Safer Shopping has been compiled to put you, the consumer, back in control of what you buy and what you put into your body. With a little bit of knowledge about how to read food labels, and up-to-date information about which additives you need to avoid, you can very easily make some simple changes to your shopping and eating habits that will reap real benefits for your whole family.

In the following pages you'll learn how to avoid products with suspect additive ingredients. Armed with this information you can greatly reduce your consumption of these chemicals and, most likely, improve your health in the process.

Chapter 1: About this book

1.1   Introduction

This book is designed to be a practical shoppers' guide that will inform consumers about the possible health risks associated with many food additives, and how to select the best, low-additive products commonly available in our major supermarkets.

It has been compiled using the most up-to-date references about food additives and is intended to give you, the consumer, the information you need to decide which additives you wish to avoid.

Not all additives are bad or harmful, so it doesn't follow that the product with the least additives is necessarily the best. *Additive Alert: Your Guide to Safer Shopping* will tell you which additives are considered harmful or suspect, and will tell you how to read the labels so you'll know what's in the products you're buying and can confidently choose the best products which do not contain harmful additives.

Imagine you are buying potato chips for a party. You may think there's very little difference across brands, but, when it comes to additives, small differences can make a very big difference to your decision. For example:

> The ingredients panel of brand A potato chips lists only one additive: *antioxidant 319*.
>
> The ingredients panel of brand B potato chips lists two additives: *antioxidant 304* and *306*.

After reading this book you'll know to choose brand B.

Why? Because antioxidant 319 is one of the nastiest food additives and should definitely be avoided, especially by children. The full name of this additive is *Tert- butylhydroquinone*, also known as *TBHQ*. It contains petroleum derived butane and is used commonly in chips, biscuits and bakery products especially as a preservative to stop the oil going rancid. It has been shown to cause cancerous changes and birth defects in animal studies, and a dose of just 5 grams is considered a fatal dose for an adult human. Lower doses of between 1 – 4 grams have been shown to cause nausea, vomiting, delirium and collapse. It is also linked reliably to adverse behaviour effects in children. Incredibly, it is still allowed in our foods. Our regulator assures us that small amounts in our foods should be safe, but it makes no sense at all to use such a cheap and nasty, potentially dangerous additive, when perfectly safe alternatives are readily available. Antioxidants 304 and 306, are two perfectly safe, readily available alternatives which have no known health risks associated with their use.

So although brand A has only one additive, it's one you most definitely want to avoid. Armed with this knowledge, most of us would choose brand B and probably decide to never eat brand A again.

After reading this book, you'll have all the information you need to decide which additives you wish to avoid. *Additive Alert: Your Guide to Safer Shopping* will tell you which additives are linked to asthma, cancer and hyperactivity. You will also learn which additives aren't recommended for children and pregnant women, and which additives are actually *prohibited* in children's foods because of their known adverse health risks. The guide also highlights additives that are *banned in other countries* because of their adverse health risks, and those not recommended for people with kidney or liver complaints.

It is not intended for this book to be viewed as a definitive scientific reference. It is primarily an information booklet and a shoppers' guide to help consumers avoid additives they don't wish to consume.

What is provided here is a compilation of current information about the known, or suspected, adverse health effects of some food additives. This information has been sourced from a range of existing credible references as cited in the references.

1.2 What this book tells you and what it doesn't

This book will not tell you which specific products to buy, and it does not recommend any particular brand over another. That is for each of us to determine depending upon our tastes, budgets and health needs.

The book only refers to additive content and doesn't rate any other nutritional considerations such as fat, salt or fibre content. Once again, these are individual concerns that vary from person to person. In some cases, for example, the "best" choice from an additive perspective may not be the best choice in relation to fat content for you. It is up to each of us to select the products overall that meet our needs best.

However, it's a general observation that those products with few or no undesirable additives tend to be the better quality choices all round. Many of the worst additives are often found in lower quality foodstuffs.

Often these additives are cheaper processing aids, or they are additives used to bulk up food or, in some cases, to improve poor flavour. So you'll find, in general, that the foods with the worst additive contents are often the poorer choices healthwise and tastewise. Still, they sometimes win out as the cheapest option.

This book will give you a basic understanding of what food additives are and what they are used for, and also the regulation of food additives in Australia.

It will explain to you how to read food labels and will reveal the loopholes in our labelling system, and how to spot hidden additives when selecting your groceries.

It will highlight for you which additives are particularly nasty and should be avoided and why.

It will also give you some practical hints about how to modify your eating and shopping habits, to significantly and easily reduce the amount of unnecessary and unsafe food additives you and your family consume every day.

If you want more details about individual additives, this book also provides you with a detailed list of all permitted additives in Australia and their potential health impacts to keep and use as a reference.

In addition, this book provides you with some very useful contacts and links for further information, if you want to know more.

Chapter 2: Food additives: what and why?

2.1 Introduction

So what exactly are food additives? A food additive isn't a food in itself, but is defined as *any substance that is added to food to achieve a technological function*. A technological function could be anything from improving colour or taste, preserving the food, preventing rancidity or improving the texture or appearance of the food.

In Australia, there are 331 food additives currently approved for use under the Australia New Zealand Food Standards Code. This joint food code is administered by a bi-national government agency named Food Standards Australia New Zealand (FSANZ). This is the same authority which controls our food labelling laws, sets residue levels for pesticides and contaminants in foods and also oversees food surveillance and food recalls where necessary.

Thankfully, many additives used in our foods are necessary and beneficial in that they stop food from decaying, prevent bacteria and other contaminants, or they genuinely improve the food in a way which is beneficial for consumers.

However, there are many other additives present in our food supply, which are used purely for cosmetic purposes or, in some cases, to fool the consumer, and, in other cases, to boost the manufacturers' profit margin.

For example:
- Vibrant colours are added to products to appeal to children.

- Flavour enhancers are used to give extra taste to otherwise tasteless products.

- Thickeners are added to make watered down products seem more substantial.

- Preservatives are spayed on fresh foods to extend the shelf life of old produce.

These types of additives are not necessary at all, but are used at the manufacturers' discretion, and are often just a means of disguising sub standard or old foods that would otherwise not taste or look appealing.

A food additive may be from a natural source such as vitamin C (additive 300), or it may be entirely synthetic and produced in a laboratory, such as buytlated hydroxyanisole (additive 320). Just because some additives are from a natural source originally does not necessarily guarantee that they are any safer than their artificial chemical cousins. Manufacturers, though, often play heavily on the term *natural* because it sounds much safer and more appealing than *artificial*.

Food additives in Australia are classified by the functions they perform. An additive may perform different functions in different products, and its function must be declared on the label. In Australia, an additive must be declared to perform a *technological function* to be permitted.

Incredibly, though, it's the *manufacturer's* discretion, not that of FSANZ, the regulatory authority, that determines what, if any, technological function is being performed.

Take, for example, green tomato sauce. This is made green by adding in the following additives:

- Curcumin 100

- Tartrazine 102 (linked to hyperactivity, migraines, skin irritations, sleep disorders)

- Brilliant Blue 133 (a suspected carcinogen, linked to hyperactivity)

It could be argued that the only "function" of making tomato sauce green is to increase the marketing appeal to kids — hardly a necessary technological function. Nonetheless, it's totally legal under the current guidelines.

2.2 The functions of food additives

The various functions that food additives perform, beneficial or cosmetic, are as follows:

Anti-caking agents

These reduce the tendency of individual food particles to adhere and clump.

Anti-foaming agents

These prevent excessive frothing or scum forming when food is boiled.

Antioxidants

These prevent oxidation, which can lead to rancidity and colour changes.

Bleaching agents

These are used to whiten flours.

Bulking agents

These contribute to the volume of food without affecting its energy content. They are often used in low-joule food where sugar is being replaced.

Colourings

These add or restore colour to foods.

Emulsifiers

These prevent oil-and-water mixtures from separating.

Firming agents, stabilisers

These maintain the uniform dispersion of substances in solid and semi-solid food.

Flavour enhancers

These enhance the existing taste or odour of a food.

Flour-treatment agents

These improve the colour or baking quality of flour and stimulate yeast activity.

Food acids

These help to maintain a constant acid level.

Glazing agents

These are used to give food a shiny appearance and/or a protective coating.

Humectants

These help to prevent food from drying out.

Mineral salts

These are added to improve texture or water-holding capacity. They can increase plumpness and help firmness.

Preservatives

These retard or prevent spoilage by inhibiting micro-organisms.

Propellants

These are used in aerosol cans to expel the contents.

Sweetening agents

These replace the sweetness normally provided by sugars without contributing significantly to the overall energy content.

Vegetable gums

These are all derived from plant sources and help improve the texture of foods.

2.3   Additive numbers

In Australia, the number codes of our food additives correlate to the food additive codes used throughout the European Union. The World Health Organisation maintains an International Numbering System for Food Additives (INS) which assigns all food additives a number. Some countries then choose to use a letter in front of the number and some do not. For example, across the EU, food additives are known as E numbers, as they all have the letter E in front of the number. In Australia and

New Zealand we do not use a letter prefix - we just use the number code.

For Example:

- MSG in Australia is labelled as 621

- MSG in the EU is labelled as E621.

Across North America most additives are similarly labelled using the INS numbers without the E prefix. The exceptions are some food colours which have alternative codes and which are still commonly used in the USA. For example, yellow colour 102 (Tartrazine) is sometimes labelled in the USA as either 102 or FD&C Yellow 5.

2.4   Additives explosion

People have been adding things to food for centuries to help colour, sweeten, preserve and improve its taste. The original food additives were natural substances such as smoke, spices, salt, sugar, vinegar and salt petre. Over time, and with the proliferation of highly refined and processed foods, more food additives have been developed and utilised by the food industry.

Not that long ago, people ate mainly fresh foods in season and cooked things from scratch. We baked cakes and biscuits and made sauces, stews and gravies. The typical western diet of today relies extensively on packaged, highly processed, highly refined foods. Consumers today are demanding more and more variety. We expect food to last and to enjoy foods that aren't local or in season. We are also demanding that food is quick, easy and even "instant" in some cases.

Such expectations can only be met through the greatly increased use of food additives, and the food manufacturing industry is happily meeting our consumer demands by pumping our foods full of more and more additives every year. As a result, we are consuming more food additives in our daily lives then ever before. More concerning is the escalating number of food additives which our children are consuming from a very early age.

Sadly, it is impossible to provide an exact estimate of the amount of food additives we eat in Australia, as our food regulator will not provide that information. However, based on overseas data, a very conservative estimate is that we Australians each eat **at least 5 kilograms** of food additives every year. This is a staggering and sobering statistic and represents a huge change in our dietary habits in a very short space of time.

Sadly, most of us have no idea what sorts of chemicals and toxins those 5 kilograms of food additives contain, nor what the potential health effects of this incredible daily combination of food additives could be.

Although the majority of food additives found in our foods today are generally regarded to be safe, a significant number are concerning. As manufacturers continue to compete for our shopping dollar, more and more food additives are being included in our food supply, and the science to guarantee their long term safety is simply not there. Over the past century, many additives have been permitted and used in our food supply and then banned as their adverse health effects later became apparent. In these cases, the adverse health effects have only been proven *after* the additive has been in circulation for a considerable time, often decades. Only then is the real health impact on humans discernable and the additive recalled.

Unfortunately, there are still numerous additives currently permitted and widely used in our food supply that are poorly tested or, in some cases, known to be harmful and which should definitely be avoided.

In relation to health, the accepted old adage used to be *"You are what you eat"*. Nowadays, however, because our foods have changed so dramatically in such a short space of time, a more appropriate saying would be *"You are what's in the food you eat"*. It is now indisputable that a healthy diet has a pivotal role to play in disease prevention and treatment, but worldwide, we are now beginning to understand just how important it is to ensure that our foods do not contain additives and contaminants which can contribute to adverse heath effects.

Let's have a look at some of the global health dilemmas confronting us all at the moment and consider the many factors which are contributing to what is now regarded as a global tsunami of ill health.

Chapter 3: Additives and health concerns

3.1   A picture of health

Consider for a moment the following snapshot of the health of our society in 2017:

Obesity

- Obesity has become our number one national health crisis and has now overtaken smoking as the leading cause of premature death in this country. We officially have an obesity epidemic in Australia, affecting both adults and children, and Australia is now ranked as one of the fattest nations in the developed world. One in four Australian children are now overweight or obese, and we are one of the few nations in the world where childhood obesity is increasing faster than adult obesity. On current trends it is estimated that half of all young Australians will be overweight or obese by the year 2025. The prevalence of obesity has more than doubled in the past 20 years and most recent research estimates that over 17 million Australians are now overweight or obese. Of most concern is the prediction that this generation of children is ***more likely to die at an earlier age than their parents***, due simply to obesity and the complications associated with this epidemic.

Diabetes

- Diabetes is the world's fastest growing chronic disease. In Australia, diabetes prevalence has increased at the rate of 8% per year since the year 2000, and diabetes is now the seventh highest cause of death by disease in Australia. Diabetes currently affects 1.8 million Australians with 275 new cases diagnosed every day. At current rates, it is estimated that by 2017 there will be 3.6 million Australians with diabetes. There are 2 types of diabetes. Type 1 is an auto immune disease which usually develops in childhood, and for which there is currently no cure. Type 2 Diabetes, or *lifestyle diabetes*, is thought to be entirely preventable by adopting a healthy diet and active lifestyle. Once regarded as an adult disease, type 2 diabetes is now affecting children worldwide at ever increasing rates, due primarily to the escalating obesity rates in children, resuting from poor diet and lifestyle choices. Diabetes is a serious disease. Consequences of diabetes include blindness, kidney failure, heart failure and amputations, not to mention premature death.

Cancer

- More kids are getting cancer every year. The incidence of brain tumours in particular has been rising steadily and this remains the most common life threatening form of tumour in children. Current estimates are that more than 1200 people die each year from brain tumours and approximately 300 children are diagnosed with brain tumours every year. The most recent research indicates that cancer rates in girls is increasing at a faster rate than in boys and the experts have no idea why. Cancer remains the biggest killer of children from disease in Australia. Cancer rates in general across the country also continue to rise and it is now estimated that 1 in every 2 Australians will develop cancer of some sort throughout their life. Cancer is the second leading cause of death for all Australians. More than 44 000 people died from cancer in 2014 and this number continues to rise every year. By 2020 it is estimated that more than 150 000 Australians will be diagnosed with cancer every year.

Bowel Cancer

- More than 14 000 Australians are told they have bowel cancer every year and it is the most frequently occurring cancer in Australia to affect both men and women. Bowel cancer rates are increasing at an alarming rate throughout the population, but the most worrying aspect of this trend is the increasing rate at which young Australians are now being diagnosed with this terrible disease. Figures from Bowel Cancer Australia reveal that the number of bowel cancer cases in people aged between 20 and 34 has increased a staggering 64 per cent over the past 20 years. Once regarded as a disease of old age, doctors are now puzzled by the alarming increase in younger and younger patients. In June 2010, the Royal Brisbane Hospital reported the youngest patient diagnosed was age 13, and that patients in their 20's, with no family history of the disease, are becoming a more common statistic.

Heart Disease
- Heart disease is still the leading cause of death in Australia. In 2015 cardiovascular disease claimed the lives of over 46 000 Australians (33% of all deaths), and these deaths were largely preventable through diet and lifestyle factors. Cardiovascular disease kills one Australian every 10 minutes. Once thought of as a disease of middle aged men, many people are unaware that this disease is now the number one killer of Australian women and is also affecting children. According to the Heart Research Institute, a staggering 40% of Australian children show early signs of artherosclerosis (thickening of the arteries) by the age of 15. This is due largely to diet and lifestyle and is entirely preventable in most cases.

Asthma
- The most recent research indicates that asthma rates in Australia have fallen over the past decade, yet we continue to have one of the highest rates in the world for this debilitating condition. It is still estimated that about 1 in 10 Australians have asthma (about 2 million people) but the incidence in children appears to have fallen significantly over the past few years from one in four (25%) to an estimated 15% of children diagnosed with chronic asthma. About half as many again are thought to suffer from regular wheezing and asthma related symptoms. Asthma is the most common cause of hospital admissions amongst Australian children. There are numerous common food additives, especially preservatives found in drinks and dried fruits, that are proven asthma triggers. Consumption of these additives is comparatively very high in Australia , especially among children, which is thought to be a significant contributing factor to our high asthma rates.

Food Allergies
- Just as we have one of the highest asthma rates in the world, Australian children also have the highest recorded rate of food allergies in the world. A 2011 study done by the Murdoch Childrens' Research Institute found that one in 10 Australian children now has a food allergy, and experts are concerned that this signals a new wave of chronic disease amongst Australian children. The reasons behind this

allergy epidemic are not understood, although diet, lifestyle and environment are thought to be the key drivers.

Autism

- Autism Spectrum Disorders (ASD) are lifelong developmental disabilities which typically manifest in children from about the age of 2. In what is now being touted as an emerging health crisis for this and future generations, autism rates in Australia and all over the world have been growing exponentially over the past 50 years. Once considered a rare condition, autism is now the fastest growing development disorder around the world. In the 1980's the prevalence of autism was estimated at 1 in every 10 000 children. Today ASD rates in Australia are estimated at 1 in every 125 children, and 1 in every 100 in New Zealand. This staggering increase can not be explained away by better diagnosis or awareness, so diet and environmental factors are believed to be the key drivers. Autism has now reached what is regarded as epidemic proportions and again, the experts don't know why this is happening or how to reverse the trend.

Mental Health

- As a nation, our mental health is also deteriorating along side our physical well being. Mental illness is the third highest burden of disease in Austraila with approximately 20% of Australians suffering from depression and this rate is steadily increasing. Each year a further 20 000 Australians are found to have a mental illness and overall, about 45% of adult Australians will experience a mental illness at some stage in their lives.

Most worrying again though, is the steadily increasing diagnosis of depression and anxiety disorders in our children and adolescents. The greatest number of people with a mental illness are within the 18 – 24 year age group. Data published in 2008 revealed that 7% of Australian children aged 0 – 17 were experiencing mental health problems, and 12% of 13 – 17 year olds reported having suicidal thoughts. Mental illness in the very young is also increasing dramatically for reasons which are not yet clear. Some studies have found that 4 in 100 preschoolers (4%) have some symptoms of depressions and it is now a well established trend to prescribe younger and younger children a variety of mood stabilising or antidepressant medications. In May 2011 Federal Health Department data revealed that prescribing rates of anti depressant drugs in children aged 2 – 6 years increased 67% in just 3 years. The government refused to release data on prescription rates for children under 2 years, so it is unknown just how many children in that age group are being treated with these drugs.

Behavioural Problems
* Previously rare behavioural problems such as Attention Deficit Disorder (ADD) Attention Deficit and Hyperactivity Disorder (ADHD), Oppositional Defiance Disorder (ODD) and Conduct Disorder (CD) continue to rise and have now become common conditions amongst school children in Australia. It is estimated that more than 350 000 Australian children and adolescents have ADHD, and that 1 in 50 children are on stimulant medications such as dexamphetamine to control their behaviour. There are very serious concerns about the long term safety of such medications in children, and of most concern, is the proven potential for these drugs to trigger suicidal tendencies in children.

Teen Suicide
* Teen suicide rates for males in Australia have quadrupled since the 1960's. One in five Australian adolescents is now estimated to have significant mental health problems. In 2016 suicide rates for young Australians hit an all time high and a third of all young male deaths in Australia are now attributed to suicide. Across the population, Australia loses seven people per day to suicide and, in 2017, more than 2000 suicide deaths are predicted. This preventable death rate exceeds the death toll every year from breast cancer and is more than 40 percent higher than the national road toll.

Dementia

- Dementia describes a collection of conditions which affect the brain, leading to loss of function and abilities. The most common forms in Australia are Alzeihmers Disease and Parkinson's disease, both conditions which have typically been associated with old age. However, incidence rates of these cruel diseases are on the increase in Australia at unprecedented levels. Dementia is now the third leading cause of death in Australia and, at current rates, it is estimated that more than 1 million Australians will have dementia by the year 2050. Of most concern is the rapid emergence of Younger Onset Dementia. Worldwide, dementia is no longer a disease of old age. People are developing dementia as young as 30. Again the reasons for this dramatic change are not well understood as yet, but environmental and dietary factors are believed to be the driving factors behind this alarming shift.

And this is the lucky country!

We *are* lucky in that we have excellent diagnosis and access to treatment options, but this is not reducing the incidence of these crippling conditions. Statistics like these are sending us a very clear message – unless something changes dramatically we are facing a fairly bleak future on the health front. What is even more alarming and indisputable is the fact that we have a *child health crisis* on our hands in Australia. We cannot ignore the grim prediction now being made by many eminent and reputable professionals that this generation of children is the first generation of children likely to die before their parents.

So what can we do? For more and more people worldwide, including an ever growing number of health professionals, the path towards arresting these alarming trends lies in prevention, not treatment of the symptoms once disease is already well entrenched. When we start to focus on prevention, this is where commonsense tells us that we need to look closely at *all* contributing factors, including diet.

3.2   So what's going on?

Many factors are contributing to the mental and physical health problems that are becoming so entrenched in our society that they are becoming normalised. For a child today to be obese, to suffer from Type 2 Diabetes, asthma or mental health problems is no longer rare or regarded as unusual, as the previous statistics clearly demonstrate.

It wasn't always this way, was it?

Think back to when you went to school. How many kids did you know with asthma? Were obese or overweight children a common sight? Sure, there were a few high-spirited ratbags in every school — the ones who were always in trouble — but was one in every five kids clinically depressed or suffering from behavioural or learning problems? It didn't seem that way to me.

Better diagnosis and community awareness of chronic conditions such as cancer, asthma, diabetes and behavioural disorders can definitely help explain some of the rising incidence of all these serious ailments. Many professionals argue, though, that it cannot *all* be put down to just better diagnosis.

So what has changed?

The answer is a lot has changed, and very quickly, but two factors in particular are most regarded as having the biggest impact on our current health.

First, our environment has changed. We are now being exposed to environmental toxins at previously unimaginable concentrations. Unless you live in a sterile bubble, you're exposed to an unbelievable cocktail of environmental toxins in every facet of your life, and have been since before you were born.

Recent studies have shown that the cord blood of new born babies is now contaminated with hundreds of toxic chemicals including heavy metals like mercury and lead, pesticides, flame retardants and household chemicals.

Samples of mother's breast milk similarly reveal significant residues of DDT and other toxic chemicals banned many years ago. These agents are known to cause cancer, deformities, physical and mental problems, and are being passed along from grandmother to mother to child. Pesticides, fertilisers, household and industrial chemicals pervade every aspect of daily lives. From the pesticide residues in food, to the toxins in the air we breathe, the water we drink and the products we use in our homes and on our bodies, it's all just one big chemical cocktail, the ongoing combination effect of which is unknown.

Second, our diet has changed dramatically in a very small space of time. The past 50 years has seen a phenomenal increase in the demand for processed and refined foods. This has led to dramatic changes to the way in which our food is grown, produced and processed and has also resulted in significant changes to the types of foods we choose to eat and feed our families. Previously, our foods were grown locally by small scale farmers and the use of pesticides, fertilisers and antibiotics was minimal, We enjoyed eating food that was locally grown and we were able to eat seasonally, so our diets were more varied. We did not routinely eat a lot of processed and packaged foods. Prior to the 1970's fast foods such as Macdonald's and the like were simply not a regular part of our diets.

Today, however, the small farmers and producers have been taken over by the large companies and our foods are grown and produced on a massive scale. As a result the routine use of pesticides, fertilisers and antibiotics has also increased drastically. Put simply, our fresh foods are now more contaminated than ever before. We also eat many more processed food products than ever before, and these new products are full of food additives, preservatives and processing aids which make then quick, convenient, long lasting and profitable. Consequently, we are all eating more food additives and getting less nutrition out of our foods, than we have ever done before.

3.3　Could it be the food?

In the 1970s, a US researcher, Dr Ben Feingold, developed a diet free of synthetic colourings, preservatives and naturally occurring salicylates that became known as the Feingold diet. It was designed to assist primarily in the management of hyperactive children, and its introduction heralded a new awareness about the link between food additives and health problems.

Since then, the debate about the effect of food additives on health has continued strongly. Ongoing research and scrutiny is showing substantial scientific and anecdotal links between the growing use of certain food additives in our over-processed diets, and the explosion of a multitude of physical and behavioural health problems in our society. As the body of research slowly continues to grow, it is becoming clearer and clearer that there are some food additives which simply should not continue to be allowed in our foods.

Here are some of the facts we currently know about some of the additives in our foods:

- Many food colourings are proven animal carcinogens and mutagens. These same additives are also known to elicit hyperactivity and behaviour problems in children.

- Many preservatives, especially the sulphites and benzoates, are known to trigger asthma in both adults and children.

- Another group of common preservatives used in bread products, the propionates, have been shown to contribute to behaviour and concentration problems in children. Most recently, research has shown a possible link between propionates and the development autism spectrum disorder symptoms in children.

- Some common antioxidants found in products like peanut butter and biscuits are definite animal carcinogens. These additives are also proven xenoestrogens – chemicals which mimic the effect of oestrogen in the body.

- Flavour enhancers are implicated in a range of serious health impacts including nausea, restlessness, skin complaints, migraines, sleeping problems, terrible rashes, behaviour and learning problems. Most recently these additives are also being queried in relation to obesity and depression, two of the biggest threats facing this generation of children.

- Serious concerns surround the long term safety of the use of a multitude of artificial sweeteners, especially their use by children. Some common artificial sweeteners are linked convincingly to kidney, bladder and pancreatic cancer, whilst others are known neurotoxins which have been shown to adversely effect the brain and developing nervous system.

- Other additives are actually prohibited in Australia by law from their use in foods intended for infants and young children, and yet, in practice, they are widely used in foods which young children eat every day.

- Finally there are some additives which are known to cross the placenta and which may cause damage in utero. These additives are not recommended for pregnant women.

3.4   Food allergies and food intolerance

When we talk about "having a reaction to food additives" no one is suggesting that the food you buy in the supermarket containing colours and preservatives will make you keel over instantly or trigger a violent and obvious reaction. What more and more people are coming to understand though, is that it is the long term , cumulative, chronic effects of these food additives in our diets which we need to be aware of and concerned about.

It can be very difficult to accept the notion that small amounts of additives in our foods can really be implicated in serious ailments such as asthma, migraines, eczema, insomnia, depression and behaviour problems. However, since Dr Feingold's work in the 1970's, science has come a very long way. Every year, more and more reputable data is confirming that the additives in our foods, can and do, have a very real impact on mental and physical health, in both adults and children.

Not everybody is affected by food additives in the same way, and, for reasons which are not yet well understood, sensitivities vary greatly. Some people are exquisitely sensitive to some food additives. There are many adult asthmatics who will testify to the fact that just one or two dried apricots will guarantee them an imminent asthma attack. Similarly, there are many people who can not enjoy takeaway food because they know that the smallest amount of added monosodium glutamate (MSG) will cause them a migraine, sleepless night or a trip to hospital with heart palpitations. At a child's party we can observe that some children seem to be able to eat brightly coloured lollies with no obvious or immediate adverse effects. For many others however, to eat the same lollies will inevitably lead to tears, tantrums and a sharp decline in their behaviour and emotional control.

What the most recent science is telling us though, is that more and more people are developing sensitivities to food additives and chemicals, and these intolerances manifest in many different ways. Unfortunately though, most people are unaware that their overall physical and mental health may be impacted by the common side effects of many food additives in the foods they eat. Equally, most people are unaware that their family's health and general well being could be greatly improved by the removal of common food additives from their diet.

Food Intolerance is the term used to describe reactions to food additives as well as reactions to natural chemicals in food such as gluten in wheat or lactose sugar in dairy products. These types of reactions are also on the rise within the community alongside an increasing prevalence of intolerance reactions to food additives.

Whilst an accurate estimate of how many people are affected by food intolerance is not currently available, what we do know is that every year the numbers are increasing rapidly for two reasons. Firstly, more and more people are coming to understand that food intolerance may be contributing to their symptoms, usually after a long process of trial and error and diet experimentation. Chronic ailments and symptoms previously put down to environment, genetics or just bad luck are now being successfully managed and alleviated through diet and lifestyle modifications.

Secondly, our over exposure to chemicals and toxins in both our environment and food, is causing more and more people – especially children – to become over-sensitised, and this is manifesting in rapidly rising numbers of people with food additive and other chemical sensitivity problems.

Food intolerance is very different to food allergy and can be difficult to understand, but it is a very real and growing problem worldwide. True food allergies are also on the rise worldwide, and, in this generation of children, we are seeing an escalating rate of potentially fatal food allergies such has never before been seen. A recent study estimated that 1 in 10 Australian children suffer from a food allergy, one of the highest published rates in the world. Australia is regarded as being on the verge of a food allergy epidemic, and the experts have no idea why this is happening or how to stop it.

True food allergies are able to be accurately diagnosed and measured as they involve a true immune response. Food allergies trigger an adverse response to a food protein that the body mistakenly believes is harmful. The immune system then releases massive amounts of chemicals, triggering symptoms that can affect a persons breathing, gastrointestinal tract, skin and heart. If left untreated, food allergy reactions can be fatal. There is no known cure for true food allergy. Common food allergens are peanuts, soy, shellfish, nuts, milk, eggs and fish although over 170 foods have been documented to trigger true food allergy reactions.

Food intolerance however, is a complex subject and can be much harder to indentify and diagnose in the first place, as it does not involve a measurable immune response by the body. Food intolerance reactions can be many and varied and can be triggered by food additives and/or natural chemicals in food. Reactions can be delayed and very subtle, manifesting as chronic, lingering conditions such as skin disorders, headaches, sinus complaints, sleep disturbances, weight control issues, behavioural problems, and gastric complaints that sufferers often just get used to living with, unaware that food intolerance may be the underlying reason for their ongoing discomfort or problems.

Food intolerance is definitely dose related which, is why the effects of food additive intolerance is often so much easier to see in young children – they often react more quickly and more obviously than adults whose symptoms may build up slowly over time. Young children are also far more susceptible to food additive intolerance as, dose for weight, they consume far more food than adults do. Food intolerance is strongly associated with behaviour, learning and emotional control problems, as well as varied and complex physical symptoms.

For many families just gaining an awareness and understanding that intolerance to food additives can have such a far reaching effect on health and behaviour is life changing. Simply by avoiding known problem additives many people find that they see great improvement in a variety of areas, especially behaviour and concentration, sleeping issues, asthma, sinus and skin problems like eczema. For many though, discovering that reactions to food additives have been contributing to their health and behaviour problems is just a starting point, as many people who react to food additives, will also go on to discover that they may be intolerant to some natural food chemicals as well.

Food intolerance reactions to food additives and natural food chemicals can be a very complex issue to get your head around, but well worth the effort if these sorts of problems are impacting the health and wellbeing of your family. If you eliminate problem food additives but still suspect there may be a reaction to natural food chemicals, then it is best to undertake a properly supervised elimination diet with the support of a suitable dietician or naturopath familiar with food intolerance issues.

For more information on Food Intolerance and Eliminiation Diets please refer to the Food Intolerance Network via their excellent website at **www.fedup.com.au**

Chapter 4: Your health, your choice

The important issue to understand is that food intolerance and the effects of food additives are not just an issue for those with chronic health ailments, colicky babies, hyperactive kids or children with behavioural problems. These are the more obvious reactions in those people who react to lower doses, but we are all consuming these additives in ever increasing amounts. A great many people are being adversely affected by the additives in their foods everyday, but are yet to make the connection.

Just because these additives don't appear to cause an immediate effect in ourselves, doesn't mean there's no effect. What effect is being had on the inside? What will the cumulative effect be on our bodies in 15 or 20 years time?

Many people are only aware of the most obvious, well-known effects of food additives. Parents often comment about kids going "hyper" after red cordial or a junk-food binge at birthday parties, but most don't regard these effects as a serious health impact. If parents knew that the colours, preservatives and flavour enhancers that elicit these behavioural changes are also, in many cases, carcinogens, mutagens and neural toxins that may cause long-term adverse effects on their children's health, many would be appalled.

For example, because I know that yellow colour 110 (Sunset Yellow) has been proven in scientific studies to cause cancer in animal studies, I make a conscious decision not to eat it and definitely make sure I do not feed it to my children. This colour has also been proven to elicit hyperactivity in children as well skin rashes, allergic reactions and asthma in adults and children. Most recently, in 2012, this colour was identified by researchers at Newcastle University as a *xenoestrogen* – a chemical which can mimic the effect of oestrogen in the body. Clearly, this is an additive which we should not be feeding to our children, and yet it is commonly used in a huge array of products including juices, icecreams, cordials, biscuits, yoghurts, custards, rice crackers and crisps.

Most people, and all parents I am sure, would not willingly choose products containing additives such as this for their family if they were given the choice. The sad fact is though, that most people simply have no idea at all that these additives are not good for us or our children.

A growing number of people are aware of safety concerns about food additives and make an effort to steer clear of the most obvious suspects such as bright colours, MSG and artificial sweeteners. What many people don't realise is the unbelievable proliferation of less obvious, but equally harmful, additives throughout our food.

Once it was mainly the obvious junk and fast foods that contained the worst suspect additives, but the use of these additives in everyday "healthy" foods is becoming solidly entrenched.

Preservatives, colours and flavour enhancers are commonly found in margarines. Aspartame is being put in sausages and yoghurts, and chocolate biscuits are made beautifully brown by the use of red, blue, yellow and green colours. Every day it's getting harder and harder to avoid food additives as their use becomes more and more widespread.

Most people don't want to know all the details; they just want to know what's safe and what's not. Unfortunately, it's not always that easy, but the bottom line is this: *many additives in use in our foods today are, at least questionable and, at worst, known to be toxic.*

As consumers, we cannot rely on regulating authorities and especially not food manufacturing companies to safeguard our health. They both have too many vested interests — the most obvious one being money.

History has shown that many additives have previously passed laboratory tests and been permitted, only to be recalled and banned years later as obvious adverse effects in humans became apparent. Food scientists estimate that it takes about 30 years to properly monitor and evaluate the effects of a new additive in circulation in the human population. Many people are now choosing not to be the unwitting guinea pigs in these tests. Many additives are poorly tested and more information is needed, but there's enough information around today for us all to become empowered and make sensible choices about the food we eat.

As parents, it's even more important to know which additives need to be avoided and to keep these out of our children's diets as much as possible. Children need good nutrition and clean environments to allow them to develop physically, mentally and emotionally in the way that nature intended. They don't need daily doses of chemicals, stimulants and toxins.

Generally people don't want to be strictly puritan about the food they eat unless they have to, and sadly, most people will not make serious diet changes until their health is already impacted. The good news is it really isn't that hard to take control. By gaining a little bit of knowledge and shopping wisely, you can make some very significant, very smart changes to the foods you eat and the foods you avoid. These can greatly enhance the health of yourself and your family.

So much is not known about the effect of chemicals and additives in our food. Those wanting to promote additives will discredit research that shows adverse effects in animals, saying that animal tests don't necessarily translate to humans. Those on the other side of the fence will argue that any adverse effects in animals must be interpreted as being relevant to humans as a precautionary measure.

The reality is that it's up to each of us to make our own decisions and choices about the food we eat. What we should remember though, is that even if these suspect additives can never be proven to cause the ill effects in humans that they cause in animal studies, they will never be proven to be doing us any good.

> Good, fresh, real food does us good, and that is what we should be trying to eat.

Chapter 5: Regulation in Australia

The use of food additives in Australia is governed by the Food Standards Code and regulated by Food Standards Australia New Zealand (FSANZ). Their charter is to protect the health and safety of the people of Australia and New Zealand by maintaining a safe food supply.

The standard mantra in relation to food additives, from the Federal Minister down, is "If it's approved for use in Australia then it's safe". This is the stock standard response you will get if you ring FSANZ and ask any questions about the safety of any food additive currently approved for use in Australia.

In my initial research into this matter I had numerous discussions with well meaning and helpful staff at FSANZ, but I was unable to get any satisfactory answers to my questions. For example:

(My questions are shown below in bold. FSANZ responses are shown in italics.)

Why in Australia do we have additives that are prohibited in other countries as suspected or known carcinogens?

Different countries have different approval systems. Some countries ban products if they cause DNA changes at any level in any animal ... just because something causes cancer in rats and mice doesn't mean it will cause cancer in humans...

Can you provide me with a list of food additives that have been previously permitted and subsequently withdrawn because of health and/or safety concerns?

No. We don't have a database with that sort of safety information on it. There is no way of collating that sort of information–some additives have been recalled in the past for a variety of reasons but you can't get a list of them...

Can you tell me if there are any health or safety concerns associated with any permitted food additives?

No. Anything which is approved for use in Australia, is considered safe, so we cannot provide any information about any supposed safety concerns. If it's approved, it's safe ...

But what about something like Amaranth (123) — a banned carcinogen in the US that's still permitted in Australia?

The US has a different system — all additives permitted in Australia are considered safe whether or not they are banned overseas. I can't comment on other countries' systems...

Why, if some additives are prohibited in foods for infants and young children, are they present in foods such as chips, corn chips and cheese snacks, which are directly marketed at the children?

By definition, FSANZ regards infants and young children as under 12 months. Therefore, additives such as 621 and 635 are permitted in these foods, as they are not regarded as foods, which would be expected to be marketed directly to, or consumed by those under 12 months....

I have heard a statistic that we Australians each eat about 5 kilograms of food additives every year. Can you tell me if that is true or give me some statistics on this matter?

We don't have an estimate figure of the total food additive intake by Australians, nor do we know any other organisation that does, especially as annual analysis of the amount of additives eaten by individuals would not be useful as all additives approved in the food code are considered to be safe.

☙

It seems that FSANZ isn't interested in any discussion about the safety or potential adverse health effects of food additives: "*If it's approved, it's safe*". In other words, "Don't you worry about that. We're here to look after you".

Unfortunately, after my attempts to inform myself via FSANZ, I was not reassured. I was very worried.

It is not acceptable that we have additives in our food that are recognised internationally as suspected or known carcinogens. These additives are banned in other countries, or widely linked to other serious adverse health impacts, yet FSANZ permits them in our food.

Similarly, it is just plain wrong that that FSANZ continues to allow the use of food colours which have been proven to cause hyperactivity and behavioural problems in children, despite the fact that they have been withdrawn from all food across the whole European Union due to safety concerns. How can it be okay for Australian children to be exposed to these chemicals in their everyday food while European children are safeguarded?

I had always assumed that Australia would be one of the more progressive countries in matters such as this. Didn't you? Well, incredibly, this isn't so.

I had also assumed that the regulatory authority would be the best place to locate up-to-date, accurate information about food additives and their effects.

Wrong again.

Although I'm sure FSANZ has lots of up-to-date information about the known and potential effects of food additives, apparently this isn't data that they are willing to give to us, the consumers.

From my research, it appears that most Australians are unaware of the shortcomings of our regulatory body. Most people quite righty assume and expect that our food regulatory authority is regulating stringently on behalf of the Australian population. Unfortunately, it seems that FSANZ is not able to meet this basic and very reasonable expectation when it comes to keeping questionable and harmful additives out of our foods.

It is not just in the area of food additives that FSANZ are failing in their duty either. FSANZ is also responsible for labelling laws, the regulation of Genetically Modified foods and other similarly controversial areas. Sadly, just as FSANZ appears to be more concerned with protecting the interests of manufacturers over the rights of consumers in relation to food additives, their stance taken in relation to some of these other areas is worrying indeed from a consumer's perspective.

Despite strident campaigning from consumer groups such as Greenpeace and the Australian Consumers Association, FSANZ still refuses to insist on the compulsory labelling of all genetically modified content in foods. The existing legislation is fraught with loopholes and exemptions, resulting in a huge array of GM products making it onto our supermarket shelves and into our trolleys everyday. Under current laws products such as baby formula, bread, cooking oils, margarines, baked goods, biscuits, cakes and takeaway foods can all get away with not declaring GM content on their labels. If you currently think you don't eat GM foods, you may need to think again and do some detective work to find out the truth!

You may want to try it for yourself and see what level of information you can access from FSANZ to help you make informed decisions about what's really in the foods you eat.

Their contact details are listed in *Appendix 3: Useful contacts.*

Chapter 6: Testing and approval of additives

6.1   The current system

FSANZ's standard response to any query about the safety of food additives has been that all additives are stringently tested before being allowed in Australia, and are only allowed in levels considered safe. This may be true, but is it good enough? Unfortunately, what is considered safe isn't a universal concept, and the regulation of and attitudes towards food additives varies from country to country.

Before an additive can be approved for use in food in Australia there's a standard application-and-approval process set out by FSANZ. This includes (amongst many other criteria) a requirement that the *manufacturers* provide new or existing scientific evidence to demonstrate the safety of the additive. This information is evaluated — *but not conducted by* —FSANZ scientists, and the additive is subsequently allowed or denied.

Generally, additives are tested initially in two-species animal studies to see if there are any effects on DNA, any links to cancer, major damage to vital organs etc. If any signs of cellular damage (or other untoward effects) are seen at high doses then a *no-observable-effect level* is determined. This is the largest level of additive that has no noticeable effect. An *acceptable daily intake* (ADI) level for people is then set. This is expressed as a dosage per kilogram of body weight, and the quantity of additive likely to be eaten by the vast majority of people must be kept below this acceptable daily intake.

Some additives for which no harmful effects are known have no ADI set, so manufacturers can use these additives in any proportion. Others have very low ADI levels. This indicates that adverse effects were observed in the initial testing on the additive, but the ADI level represents the level of consumption, which is considered safe.

For example, Annatto (160b) has a very low ADI of 0.065 milligrams per kg of body weight, as there are still ongoing queries over the long-term safety of this additive; whereas, beta carotene (160a) has no ADI set as there are no known adverse effects associated with this additive.

6.2   So what's the problem?

There are many shortcomings with the current system of testing, approval and review of additives in Australia. With our current system, additives can be known to cause serious adverse effects at high doses in animal studies, yet small doses throughout our food are considered safe.

There are many additives which have previously been banned in other countries because of established links to adverse health impacts including cancer, but which continue to be permitted in Australia at these "safe levels". This is despite the action of other food regulators internationally which have, based on safety studies, deemed them "unsafe" and regulated to keep them out of the food supply. In many other countries, including the USA, a far more stringent "precautionary" approach is taken, especially in relation to cancerous changes demonstrated in animal studies.

The concepts of safe levels and acceptable daily intake are questionable too. These are set based on the projected average adult intake. There is no separate ADI set for children, so dose for weight, our kids are getting a much higher dose of these additives than would be intended. Also, many of the more suspect toxic additives with the lowest ADIs are found prolifically in children's foods such as lollies and snack foods. It is doubtful whether the dietary mapping done to set the ADI for general adult consumption would properly reflect what children today are really eating.

There are numerous studies demonstrating the much higher sensitivity to chemical carcinogens of young animals compared to adults. This is due to their limited physiological capability to detoxify carcinogens because of their immature liver enzymes, plus the fact that their cells are dividing more rapidly than adults, increasing the risk of DNA mutations in the cells and the development of delayed cancers in adult life.

The increased susceptibility of infants and young children to a wide range of carcinogens has been fully recognised for well over two decades, but this isn't reflected in the determination of ADI levels for additives with proven carcinogenic potential.

Additives are only tested for major physical changes, they aren't tested for neurological impacts and their effects on learning and behaviour. In the 1970s Dr Feingold wrote *"the time honoured idea that synthetic additives can be judged simply from routine carcinogenic and mutagenic standards is out of date and dangerous … "*. Well it's even more out of date now and getting more dangerous as time marches on and nothing changes.

Similarly, additives are only tested in isolation. They are not routinely tested in any combination with other additives, which is obviously how they are consumed in real life. There is no knowledge about how these additives react with each other or the long-term cumulative effect of these innumerable combinations in our system.

It is very easy for the average Australian eating a normal healthy balanced diet to consume a combination of more than 100 different additives every day, If you find this hard to believe have a look at *Chapter 12.2 Additive consumption comparison,* and ask yourself how many different additives are you and your family eating everyday?

What little independent research into the combination effects of additives that has been done is extremely alarming. In December 2005, results published from a study conducted by the University of Liverpool into the combination effect of 4 common additives set some serious alarm bells ringing. The researchers of this study examined the toxic effect on nerve cells using a combination of four common additives – aspartame, brilliant blue, msg and quinoline yellow. They discovered that the damage each additive caused was significantly greater when the additives were eaten in combination – which of course is exactly how they are eaten in real life!

The study used additives in concentrations that theoretically reflected the amount of additives which would enter the bloodstream after a typical children's snack, and they found that the additives ***stopped the nerve cells growing and interfered with the proper signalling systems.*** What is so worrying about this study is that the type of foods these additives are found in, and the amounts they are talking about, is what would be in a typical snack such as a choc milk and rice crackers, or a cordial and chips.

Thankfully, however, with research such as this emerging, there is a burgeoning awareness within the scientific and medical communities that demonstrable links between diet and medical health can be identified and that these links must be investigated. In 2004, the Telethon Institute for Child Health Research in Perth, WA, instigated a study into the relationship between junk-food diets and depression. The research has been motivated by the worrying five-fold increase in depression among Australia's young people in recent years.

Astoundingly, though, there's currently no facility through FSANZ or any other government body for consumers to report or complain about adverse health effects they experience with food additives. FSANZ acknowledges that adverse reactions do occur in a small percentage of the population and recommends that such people avoid problem additives by reading labels. They don't see it as their role though to collect any information about adverse health effects.

What is so incredible about this complete lack of interest from FSANZ, is that there *is* such a mechanism for the reporting of adverse effects of agricultural and veterinary chemicals through the *Australian Pesticides and Veterinary Medicines Authority.* It would seem that our authorities are more interested in the health of the nation's livestock than its people.

Finally, food additives are tested on animals, not humans, and the relevance of animal results will be debated depending upon which side of the fence you sit. History has shown though, that many additives have passed laboratory tests and been approved for human consumption, but have afterwards been banned as more research and the actual effect on humans came to light. The following quote sums up exactly why we should be adopting the precautionary approach when it comes to the safety of our food:

What we know:

- Every known human carcinogen causes cancer in animals.

- Every chemical known to cause brain damage in humans causes damage to the brain and nervous systems of animals.

- Every chemical known to interfere with reproductive function in humans interferes with reproductive function in animals.

- Almost every known cause of birth defects in humans also causes defects in animals.

- And, with few exceptions, when toxic chemicals harm animals, they almost always cause similar harm in humans.

**Centre for Childrens' Health and the Environment
Mount Sinai School of Medicine**

Chapter 7: Understanding labels

7.1   Introduction

Now that we know that there are many suspect additives permitted legally in our food, at least we can read the labels and choose to avoid them if we want to. Right?

Wrong.

The labels don't always tell the full story. There are several loopholes in our labelling system that can frustrate the attempts of the most dedicated consumer to make informed choices about what they eat.

Despite successive food labelling reviews undertaken by FSANZ over the years, the food labelling legislation standard in Australia is still woefully inadequate when compared to standards enjoyed by consumers in other western countries.

A major review was undertaken by FSANZ in 2002, which did achieve some modest gains for consumers in relation to nutrition panels. The most recent review was commissioned by FSANZ in 2009. This review was completed in 2011 with the publication of the report titled *Labelling Logic* and, as at May 2017, the recommendations of this review have all been implemented by FSANZ.

Despite extensive and expensive consultation around the country, final recommendations were a big disappointment to consumers. Once again, FSANZ failed to listen to consumers on matters such as food additives, GM content, nanotechnology and irradiated foods. More than 6000 individual consumers lodged submissions on these issues, yet the final recommendations failed to take any notice of the repeated call from consumers for transparent labelling of these components in our foods. The review did recommend some improvements to the labelling requirements in relation to country of origin and nutrition and health claims, but did not really result in any major gains for Australian consumers. These reviews are extremely expensive and it is unlikely that another one will be commissioned by

FSANZ for at least another 10 years. What that means for us as consumers is, between now and then, we certainly can not rely on the food labels to be telling us the complete and honest story about what is really in our foods.

Put simply, our standard of food labelling in Australia is just not good enough. In 2017, our food code and labelling laws are still riddled with loopholes and inadequacies which favour the manufacturers' interests over the rights and concerns of the consumers. These loopholes exist because of industry pressure, are driven by profit and, despite ongoing consumer campaigns, there is no indication at present of any willingness by FSANZ to adopt a more consumer friendly, precautionary stance when it comes to the labelling of our foods.

7.2 Numbers or names?

Under the current food labelling laws, manufacturers now have the choice of listing additives by either their number or their name. This means consumers have to be familiar with *both* the numbers and names to be able to decipher labels. It would have been a simple matter to legislate that manufacturers list both on their labels, but the manufacturers won out on this one. Manufacturers like to have the choice of which one to use as market research shows that consumers can be put off by too many chemical names.

For example, preservative 385 may be less confronting on your tinned crab meat than *calcium disodium ethylene-diaminetetracetate*, and flavour enhancer 635 sounds a lot more appetising in your packet soup than *disodium 5 ribonucleotides*.

7.3 The 5% loophole

With the recent changes in the labelling laws, FSANZ had the opportunity to bring in legislation to oblige manufacturers to list *all* the ingredients in their products, no matter how small the quantity, but they didn't. Once again, the pressure from the food manufacturers won out over the rights and protection of consumers' interest.

Under the laws at the moment there's what is known as *the 5% loophole*. This gaping hole in the legislation means that manufacturers can get away with not listing additives if they are present in an ingredient that comprises *5% or less of the product.*

Antioxidants in vegetable oil are the most common example of this that I have found. Many products have vegetable oil as an ingredient, and the oil will also contain antioxidants. Some of these antioxidants (such as 310, 319 or 320) are associated with adverse health impacts, but these antioxidants aren't listed if the amount of vegetable oil in the product is less than 5% of its weight.

Often, suspect additives aren't declared on labels under the protection of this loophole. Manufacturers can list compound ingredients such as margarine and breadcrumbs, and not list what is in *those* ingredients if they make up less than 5% of the final product. These ingredients often contain suspect antioxidants, colours and preservatives, but this will not be declared on the label.

Prior to December 2002, the 5% loophole was the 10% loophole. Why FSANZ bothered to change the law from 10% to 5%, rather than just get rid of the loophole altogether, is incomprehensible from a consumer's point of view.

You can find out more about what the labels won't tell you in *Chapter 8: Labelling licence: what you need to know.*

7.4   No warnings

Despite the well-recognised adverse effect of some additives on health, FSANZ don't entertain the notion of warnings on foods. Many preservatives, especially the sulphites and nitrites, are well known to be associated with asthma attacks, and yet these are added widely to fresh and processed foods with no warnings. These preservatives are sometimes added to fresh meat, especially mince and sausages, and even to fresh fish, but the consumer has no entitlement to a warning under the current laws.

There are also many additives that are *specifically banned in foods intended for infants and young children* because of their proven adverse health impacts. This, in effect, just keeps them out of infant formula and baby food, yet FSANZ is quite happy for these same additives to be widely used in foods developed and marketed fairly and squarely at older children. For some reason it's deemed perfectly safe to feed these additives to children *over* one, yet they are prohibited and considered dangerous in foods for children *under* one. A warning on these foods that they contained additives not recommended for consumption by young children would no doubt have a dramatic effect on the sales of such foods. These include some two-minute-noodle snacks, chips, rice crackers, most sausages, frankfurts and savoury biscuits.

Many colours used widely in children's food and drink products in Australia are also not subject to warning labels, despite the fact that other countries insist on warning labels. Across the entire EU, legislation enacted in 2010 demands that any product containing colours 102, 104, 110,122, 124 or 129 must display a prominent warning label stating: "***Warning: May have an adverse effect on attention and activity in children***". Our food regulator refused to follow the lead of the European food regulator on this matter and act to bring in labelling laws. As a result, these additives continue to appear in our everyday favourite foods such as milk drinks, ice creams and biscuits and most people have no idea that this unacceptable double standard exists

Despite introducing much stricter nutritional labelling, FSANZ still resists any move towards labelling of suspected carcinogenic additives in food. (After all, if it's approved, it's safe according to FSANZ.) Food labels tell us how much salt, sugar, fat and carbohydrates are in 100 grams of every product, but they don't mention the presence of potential carcinogens. If warnings declaring the presence of any known or suspected carcinogenic additives were mandatory, I am sure that consumers would vote loudly with their shopping dollars and avoid these products in droves.

Chapter 8: Labelling licence: what you need to know

8.1   Reading ingredient labels

There isn't too much to understand when it to comes to reading ingredient labels. It's more important to know how to read between the lines and recognise what's *not* on the label.

Under current laws, manufacturers must list the ingredients on all packaged foods, except if it's made and packaged on the premises (such as bread from a bakery), or if it's packaged in the presence of the customer (such as meat or cheese from a delicatessen or take-away food shop).

When reading ingredient labels, the ingredients are listed in decreasing weight, so the first ingredient listed is the largest component in the food. Additives must be listed by name or number, and by the purpose they perform in the product.

The following is an example of a label for a vegetable extract sandwich spread:

Ingredients: Vegetable Protein Extract, Sugar, Yeast Extract, Water, Colour (Caramel 150c), Salt, Cornflour, Glucose Syrup, Onion, Emulsifier (Glycerol Monostearate), Thickener (Modified Cornstarch), Food Acid (Citric), Vitamins (Niacin, Thiamin, Riboflavin), Vegetable Gum (Carrageenan), Flavour Enhancers (627,631), Spice Extract

---

From reading this label we can learn that the main ingredient is *vegetable protein extract*. This is a less concentrated form of MSG but one which is linked with the same adverse health effects of MSG. It also contains another ingredient, *yeast extract*, which again, is another dose of a less concentrated form of MSG.

It also contains the artificial colour *caramel 150c*. The safety of this additive is very questionable as it is linked to hyperactivity, gastrointestinal problems and, most recently, has been found to contain carcinogenic contaminants. *Glycerol monostearate* is an additive which is usually made from hydrogenated soya bean oil, so is almost always genetically modified in origin, but it currently has no reported adverse side effects. Similarly, *modified corn starch* and *citric acid* are regarded as generally safe additives. *Carrageenan* however, is a known animal carcinogen which caused ulcerative colitis in animal studies. Finally, *flavour enhancers 627 (disodium 5'-guanylate)* and *631 (disodium 5'-inosinate)* are both **prohibited in foods for infants and young children in Australia** and linked to many adverse reactions including asthma, rashes and hyperactivity.

Who would have thought they could fit so many nasties in one little bottle! Seriously though, many Australian children are eating sandwich spreads with ingredient lists like this every single day, and it cant be doing them good. It is also totally unnecessary with safer additives readily available to the manufacturers.

8.2   Hidden additives

Because of the 5% loophole, some additives aren't listed on the labels but are still present in the product. As previously mentioned, the most common example of this is antioxidants in vegetable oil. Most oils have some antioxidants in them. Many products now contain the safer ones 306–309, but many still use 310, 319 and 320, which are some of the worst additives linked to cancer and serious adverse health effects.

If you don't want to eat these chemicals, unfortunately the only way you can know for sure what's in these products, is to ring the company and ask what's in the oil they use.

Be on the look out for antioxidants in any products with ingredient lists that include fats such as animal oil, animal fat, butter, fat, copha, lard, milk solids, palm oil, shortening, tallow, vegetable oil, margarine. Common product lines found to contain antioxidants in oil, but not listed on the label, include biscuits, bread, spreads, soy milk drinks, cooking sauces, ice cream cones, baby food, tinned fish and frozen products such as pastries, pies, fish fingers, chicken nuggets, frozen desserts, potato products and ready meals.

8.3   No-MSG claims

Due to the bad press MSG has suffered in relation to widespread adverse health effects, many manufacturers emblazon "No MSG" messages on their packaging to attract the health conscious shopper.

Be Wary. Many, many products carrying these claims are very misleading.

Often they don't contain MSG in the form of food additive 621, but they will contain other flavour enhancers (620–635) that are associated with the same range of adverse health impacts, but are less well known. Avoid anything with flavour enhancers or hydrolysed vegetable protein if you're wanting to avoid MSG because of its health effects.

See section *9.1: MSG and flavour enhancers* for more information.

8.4   Natural colour

Many manufacturers like to use the word *natural* wherever possible to assist in marketing and to attract customers. *Natural colour* is a description often found on labels in relation to Cochineal (120), Caramel (150) and Annatto (160b).

- *Cochineal* is a red dye derived from the crushed dried bodies of pregnant scale insects which feed on cacti in Central America. An extract from the cochineal insects is combined with aluminium to form *carminic acid,* or *carmine,* known as colour 120, a very persistent pigment. This additive is associated with hyperactivity in children but, of most concern, is the increasing occurrence of true allergic reactions to this colour. Reported reactions have included urticaria (rashes), asthma, vomiting, diarrhoea, and actual anaphylaxis. It seems that just as other food allergies are increasing rapidly in the community, so are true allergic reactions to the insect protein in this " natural" dye.

- *Caramels 150(i), 150(ii), 150(iii), and 150(iv)* have nothing to do with the image of browned sugar that the name caramel conjures up. These colours are produced synthetically by the treatment of carbohydrates in the presence of chemicals such as ammonia, ammonium sulphate, sulphur dioxide and or sodium hydroxide. Once thought to only be associated with gastric upsets in some people, their overall safety is now under increased scrutiny. During the production of caramel colours, contaminants are formed and residues of these contaminants remain in the colour additives which are then added to our food and drink products. Scientific testing conducted by the National Toxicology Program in the USA in 2015 found that these contaminants were definite animal carcinogens in mice and rat models.

- *Annatto* is an increasingly commonly used colour additive which is often found in seemingly uncoloured product like, cheese, breakfast cereals, yoghurt, butter, icecream and biscuits. It is derived originally from the tropical achiote tree. Commercially the seeds of the plant are processed with solvents to extract the oil soluble dye. Annatto is associated very strongly with adverse behaviour effects in children, asthma, headaches, urticaria and true allergic reactions in rare cases.

Many food additives are derived from natural sources, but this doesn't necessarily mean that they are any safer than other additives. Be aware of this when shopping, and don't be swayed by claims of natural colours or ingredients. Natural or not, they may not be the safest choice for you.

8.5 Flavours

The use of flavours in food products isn't subject to the same laws as food additives. There are several thousand flavours permitted for use, and they don't have to be described on labels. The reason for this is that their chemical composition is too complex. A coffee flavour for example may consist of several *thousand* odorous materials, each composed of a different chemical type. This is the case for all characteristic food flavours. The bottom line is there's no way of knowing exactly what's in a flavour, so if you're concerned about additives and chemicals, it may be best to avoid all products marked *flavour added* including those labelled *nature identical flavour*.

Manufacturers do play on the perception that fruit and natural flavours are seen as healthiest by consumers, but be aware that the use of "fruit" flavours doesn't necessarily mean that there is any fruit in the product. For example, *strawberry yoghurt* must have some strawberries in it, but *strawberry flavoured yoghurt* doesn't have to contain any strawberries and may be completely artificially flavoured.

The following extract from the award winning book *Fast Food Nation* by Eric Schlosser (Penguin 2002) illustrates beautifully just how different strawberry favour is from the real thing!

> **Ingredients of a Typical "Nature Identical" Artificial Strawberry Flavour:** *Amyl acetate, amyl butyrate, amyl valerate, anethol, anisyl formate, benzyl acetate, benzyl isobutyrate, butyric acid, cinnamyl isobutyrate, cinnamyl valerate, cognac essential oil, diacetyl, dipropyl ketone, ethyl acetate, ethyl amyl ketone, ethyl butryate, ethyl cinnamate, ethyl heptanoate, ethyl heptylate, ethyl lactate, ethyl methylphenylglycidate, ethyl nitrate, ethyl propionate, ethyl valerate, heliotropin, hydroxyphenyl – 2-butanone, a-ionone, isobutyl anthranilate, isobutyl butyrate, lemon essential oil, maltol, 4-methylacetophenone, methyl anthranilate, methyl benzoate, methyl cinnamate, methyl heptine carbonate, methyl naphthyl ketone, methyl salicylate, mint essential oil, neroli essential oil, nerolin, neryl isobutyrate, orris butter, phenethyl alcohol, rose, rum, ether, y-undecalactone, vanilin and solvent.*

8.6   Organic claims

Consumers, in general, are becoming more discerning and health conscious. Manufacturers have picked up on this and compete for our shopping dollars with labelling that leaps out and attracts shoppers wanting healthier products. As a result, the terms *organic* and *all natural* are appearing more and more on labels across the complete product range.

Beware though: a product isn't organic unless it's labelled *certified organic*; and many *all natural* products do, on closer examination, contain many suspect additives, even if they are naturally sourced. Remember, *natural* doesn't necessarily mean safer.

8.7   No artificial preservatives

No artificial preservatives is another common phrase found on labels. It is designed to attract or sway shoppers' choice in favour of the product. This is often a true statement, but it doesn't necessarily mean the product is preservative free. There are many preservatives that are naturally sourced and, as with colours, *natural* doesn't necessarily mean safer, particularly for asthmatics.

8.8   Advertising by omission

This is another common ploy to fool the consumer. Manufacturers naturally want to advertise the best points of their products, not draw your attention to the less appealing aspects. After all, they want you to buy their product to help their profits.

For example, the packet of a popular cheese-flavoured snack is emblazoned with an attention grabbing:

> *No Preservatives*
>
> *No Artificial Colours*
>
> *No Artificial Flavours*

These statements are true. What they don't draw your attention to is the use of three flavour enhancers: MSG (621), *disodium guanylate* (627) and *disodium inosinate* (631). All of these additives are prohibited in foods for infants and young children and are linked to an array of adverse health effects ranging from headaches, asthma, sleep disturbance, behaviour and learning problems in children. Unfortunately, children would be the major consumers of products like this.

8.9   Customer enquiry services

If you have a query about what's in a product, you can contact the manufacturer whose contact details will be on the label. The bigger companies have toll-free numbers and specially trained staff, but many smaller manufacturers don't, so you may end up talking to the factory supervisor or someone with little or no knowledge about food additives.

Many of the larger brands are owned by the larger food manufacturing outfits such as Unilever, Goodman Fielder, etc so you may find many different brands serviced by the same customer-service centres. Supermarket home-brand lines are often actually manufactured by these big names also, so you might find, for example, that the contact number for *Coles Homebrand Fish Fingers* is the same as a *Birds Eye* product, and that the products are, in fact, identical.

From my experience researching this book, most of the customer-service staff I encountered were well meaning and helpful, some outstandingly so. A small number were not, and some were quite hostile and totally unhelpful when I explained that I wanted to know about additives because of health concerns.

Be aware that if you ring for more information on a product, that the staff answering your call may know very little if anything about the potential health impacts of food additives. The phone staff are *company trained* to promote products and reassure consumers that they should purchase their products, and they only have the information available that is provided for them by the company. Usually they operate from databases with product specifications that match the information on the labels, so they often know nothing more than you know from reading the label.

If you want to know more (for example, if there's any antioxidant in a vegetable oil which was not listed on the label), you may initially be told quite definitely that if it's not on the label, it's not in the product. Many of these staff aren't aware of the 5% loophole and will swear black and blue that their labels are accurate, only to be forced to go away and check and find out they were wrong.

Don't be afraid to insist politely that you really need to know for health reasons. Ask them to check with their suppliers, if necessary, to give you a 100% correct answer.

It is your right as a consumer to be able to find out exactly what is in the food you eat. Don't be intimidated or put off with inadequate answers and try to have the confidence to complain to a supervisor if your enquiry isn't answered adequately.

The only way consumers are going to influence manufacturers is by letting them know what we will and won't buy. If you do find out that a product has an additive you wish to avoid, make sure you tell the company representative that you'll avoid their product because of their use of unsafe additives. This type of feedback, as well as actually voting with our shopping dollars and *not* buying the products, is the only way to make the manufacturers sit up and take note.

Chapter 9: The ones to watch out for

Although a full list of all additives and their potential health effects is provided at the back of this book for your reference, the widespread and increasing use of some additives is so disturbing that they require special mention in this chapter. This way, you, the consumer, have all the necessary information to decide which additives you wish to avoid.

9.1 MSG and flavour enhancers

MSG is the sodium salt of glutamic acid. In its processed form as the food additive MSG 621, it is a white powder which looks like salt or sugar. It has no taste of its own and no nutritional value, but is used to enhance or modify flavours of foods. Most people have heard of it due to its widespread use in Chinese food and the resulting bad press of what became known as "Chinese restaurant syndrome". After eating Chinese food, some people were reporting a wide range of adverse health effects including sweating, heart palpitations, sleeplessness, heartburn, asthma, rashes, nausea and migraines. Studies have shown that while just 0.5 milligrams of MSG is enough to cause symptoms in sensitive people, some Chinese meals were found to contain up to 10 milligrams of MSG.

Discovered in Japan, MSG was not commonly added to western diets until after World War II when American food manufacturers began adding it to their products. No significant safety studies were performed and, since the 1940s, MSG usage has doubled every decade. This represents one of the most significant changes to our diets in the past 50 years.

Originally, there were no restrictions on the use of MSG in foods, but in 1969 it was prohibited from use in baby foods in the USA due to damning research demonstrating that MSG caused detrimental effects on young animals, particularly the brain and nervous systems. Pregnant monkeys fed MSG gave birth to brain-damaged offspring, and this was also found with pregnant rats.

MSG is still prohibited from use in baby foods in Australia, because of its proven ability to damage the brain and developing nervous system, but this effectively only keeps it out of infant formulas and baby food. MSG is still widely used in many foods eaten regularly by young children and pregnant women, with no warnings required on the labels.

MSG stands for *Monosodium Glutamate*, and it is the adverse effect of excess glutamate which is of concern. It is very important to understand the difference between *natural glutamate* such as that found in broccoli and cheese, and *processed free glutamate* as is found in the food additive MSG, because the glutamate industry goes to great lengths and expense to reassure consumers that MSG is safe and beneficial, when in fact there is a huge difference between the effects of natural and processed glutamate.

Glutamate is an important neurotransmitter and, in normal levels in the body, it does an important job allowing the cells in the brain to communicate with each other. However, when the brain is exposed to excessive amounts of glutamate, serious damage can occur. Glutamate belongs to a group of amino acids (including cysteine, aspartate and glutamate) which are classified as *"excitotoxins"*. Excitotoxins are substances that, when applied to neurons (brain cells) will cause them to become overstimulated and, if overstimulated too much, they will die. Put simply, too much MSG can kill our brain cells. Although this effect is a worry for anyone, it is most concerning in relation to children and pregnant women.

Low levels of glutamate in the form of MSG are found naturally in many foods such as tomatoes, broccoli, mushrooms, spinach and grapes. Unless you're truly allergic or intolerant to MSG, eating MSG at these natural levels is not a problem. In this state, the glutamate is bound to protein and is present in low concentrations, so that when we eat these foods, they are digested slowly and the glutamate is released into our bloodstream at the right concentration. The glutamate is then taken up into the brain at the right levels where it helps to perform essential functions within our bodies. Natural levels of bound glutamate like this in natural foods are not something you need to be concerned about.

However, this has got very little to do with the high levels of processed free glutamate, which is what the food additive MSG is made up of. To make the food additive MSG, the food manufacturers extract the natural glutamate from the raw ingredients, and the glutamate is processed so that it is no longer bound to protein. It is now called *processed free glutamate* – and it is highly, highly concentrated at levels that far exceed the levels found naturally in foods. When we eat artificially high doses of MSG like this, such as is found in our chips and snack foods, it is like a shot or a dose of free glutamate into our bloodstream. We end up with excessive quantities of glutamate in our system, and this is a problem.

The blood–brain barrier is a system in the walls of the capillaries within the brain that works to keep toxic substances, including excess glutamate levels, from entering the brain. However, there are parts of the brain that aren't protected by this barrier. This allows excess glutamates to enter the brain. It is also known that prolonged, high levels of excessive glutamate exposure can cause glutamates to seep through the blood–brain barrier and impact the brain.

In natural foods containing glutamate, the different amino acids compete with each other to get into the brain, so only a little of each gets in at the right concentrations. By contrast when we eat foods high in processed free glutamate, excess glutamate on its own gets in at much higher concentrations than normal, causing excitotoxic effects of the brain.

Young children are particularly at risk because the blood brain barrier is not fully developed during infancy and childhood. This allows excess glutamate to be delivered to the brain. Damage is also known to occur *in utero* as MSG has been shown to cross the placenta and concentrate in the foetus at levels twice that of the mother. It is this neurotoxic action of glutamate on the brain that is the most concerning adverse health effect linked to MSG. The effect on young children is again most worrisome because of the disproportionate dose they receive after eating foods containing extremely high levels of MSG.

Ongoing research has implicated excess glutamate as a contributing factor in learning disorders, brain tumours, hyperactivity, Parkinson's disease, Alzheimer's disease and endocrine-system problems developing later in life. MSG is also linked to asthma and a wide range of serious adverse health effects including sleep disturbances, migraine, irritability and depression.

Most recently, MSG is being implicated in the alarming obesity epidemic confronting developed countries all over the world. Research conducted in 2005 by a team of Spanish and German scientists found that when given to rats at concentrations only slightly higher than those found in human foods, MSG caused a massive 40% increase in appetite. MSG is used in foods as a flavour enhancer to make foods taste better, so it is not surprising that its use in foods leads to such dramatic overeating. Many are now linking the steadily increasing use of MSG in our foods since the 1950's to the parallel increase in obesity rates within western society. What is more concerning though is that these findings are nothing new. Studies done as far back as 1968 first identified that MSG induced obesity in animal studies.

Because the damaging effect of MSG on the developing brain is so well documented, many researchers are now wondering if this exponential increase in MSG consumption is also a major contributing factor to the increased levels of depression, violence, behavioural and learning disorders evident in western societies around the world today. In January 2005 British researchers reported that changes in diet over the past fifty years appear to be an important factor behind a significant rise in mental ill health. Research has also confirmed that MSG has an alarming effect on anger. Studies done as far back as 1979 revealed that MSG exposure was able to produce intense rage reactions in animal subjects.

With so much evidence confirming that MSG is able to produce such serious detrimental effects, it is of great concern that the use of this food additive is becoming so wide spread that it is becoming very difficult to avoid it without a concerted effort. This generation of children are eating worrying amounts of MSG and their exposure is beginning before they are born via their mothers' diet. What is of even more concern is the knowledge that humans are the most susceptible to physical damage from ingested MSG. According to Professor Russell Blaylock, author of *Health and Nutrition Secrets That Can Save your Life*, humans possess a sensitivity to MSG five times greater than that of the mouse and twenty times greater than the rhesus monkey.

The evidence is clear that MSG causes damage to animals. Why on earth are we continuing to consume this toxin in our foods?

9.2 Avoiding MSG isn't as easy as it should be

In response to the growing concern and awareness about the adverse effects of MSG, food manufacturers and the glutamate manufacturers have joined together to form a special lobby group called *The Glutamate Association* to counter any negative claims about MSG. This group has an obvious vested interest in keeping MSG and other flavour enhancers on the market and in keeping information off food labels.

As we have seen, manufacturers can list additives either by name or by a number and the function they perform. MSG is often not on the label, but is instead identified as *flavour enhancer 621*, which isn't so readily recognisable. Alternatively, and increasingly common, they use other glutamates and flavour enhancers such as 620, 622, 623, 624, 625, 627, 631 and 635. These aren't as well known to consumers. These other glutamates are all linked to the same adverse health impacts as MSG, while 627, 631 and 635 are known to cause other serious adverse health effects.

The use in particular of flavour enhancer 635 (*disodium 5 ribonucleotides*) has only been permitted in Australian foods for the past five years, yet it is making its presence known loudly. It has been linked with a wide range of adverse effects including sleep disturbance, skin complaints and the appearance of a distinctive, unbearably itchy rash known as *ribo rash*. The adverse effects of this additive are becoming so common that the Royal Prince Alfred Hospital Allergy Unit commissioned a clinical study in 2003 to investigate the complaints.

Concern about the use of MSG and other similar additives is a global issue. In June 2003 it was reported that the Education Ministry in Thailand banned the use of MSG in school canteen meals along with other harmful additives. If officials in Thailand are sufficiently concerned about the health impacts of these additives, it begs the question why aren't regulators here in Australia?

9.3 Ways to disguise MSG in foods.

Today, hundreds of thousands of tonnes of MSG are produced and added to foods that we eat. An additive that used to be found mainly in Chinese and very spicy foods and was eaten infrequently is now so widespread it's getting difficult to avoid.

It is found in most snacks and savoury biscuits, sauces and condiments, preserved and "fresh meats" (including bacon, polony, ham and sausages), many tinned savoury foods, packet soups, frozen meals and packaged meals, and even in some margarines.

As consumers are becoming more wary of MSG, manufacturers are cleverly using other non-regulated ingredients that also contain high levels of processed free glutamate, but which are not pure MSG, to avoid having to list MSG on their labels. These ingredients allow manufacturers to still get the MSG effect on the flavour of their product, but these ingredients are still high in the excitotoxic processed free glutamate.

One of the most common ingredients used as a substitute for MSG is *Hydrolysed Vegetable Protein*. This healthy sounding ingredient is commonly found in many products which quite legally promote themselves as being MSG free. What the labels will neglect to mention is the fact that the product is loaded with another form of highly concentrated processed free glutamate, which you now know to have the same adverse effects as MSG.

In his book *Excitotoxins: The Taste That Kills*, Dr Russell Blaylock (a Professor of Neurosurgery at the Medical University of Mississippi), lists the following common sources of concentrated processed free glutamate (MSG) which are often included in foods but not labelled as MSG:

Additives that always contain MSG

monosodium glutamate *potassium glutamate*
*hydrolysed vegetable protein *** *hydrolysed protein*
hydrolysed plant protein *autolysed yeast*
plant protein extract *sodium caseinate*
calcium caseinate *yeast extract*
hydrolysed oat flour *textured protein*
hydrolysed (anything else)

Additives that frequently contain processed free glutamate (MSG)

malt extract *malt flavour*
bouillon *broth*
stock *flavouring*
natural flavouring *spices*
natural beef or chicken flavour *seasoning*

Dr Blaylock provides this explanation of what exactly this healthy sounding ingredient really is.

Hydrolysed vegetable protein

Hydrolysed vegetable protein is a concentrated form of natural MSG that is now often used by manufacturers instead of MSG as a way around consumer concern. Often, products with high amounts of HVP boldly market themselves as "MSG free" to attract consumers who are unaware that HVP contains high concentrations of glutamates and has the same health effects as MSG.

HVP is made from junk vegetables selected for their high quantity of excitotoxins; e.g. glutamate. The vegetables are boiled in a vat of sulphuric acid for several hours then the acid is neutralised with caustic soda. The brown sludge is scraped off the top and dried into a powder. The powder contains known carcinogens and dicarboxylic acid, the safety of which is unknown. MSG is often added to this powder. Finally, the powder is put in our food, including baby food, and we eat it.

So, avoiding MSG isn't always that easy. Luckily most people aren't truly allergic to MSG. If you are, though, you'll need to avoid all products that have any of the above ingredients.

If you want to avoid MSG because of the concerning adverse effects, you'll need to decide how far you want to take it. It can be very limiting to avoid all food with *flavour* or *seasoning* as an ingredient, but the facts are that there is no way of knowing exactly what is in these ingredients.

Depending on your health and motivation, you may just choose to avoid the main sources and not buy anything with flavour enhancers **620–637** or hydrolysed vegetable protein on the label. By adopting a simple change like this, you'll be making a very significant improvement to your overall health and wellbeing.

9.4   Aspartame and artificial sweeteners

Aspartame is another food additive that is becoming increasingly commonplace in the foods we buy. It is also associated with a concerning array of adverse health effects. Most people assume that Aspartame and artificial sweeteners are only used in diet foods and drinks and, as such, many of us aren't aware that we're consuming these additives.

Like MSG, the use of Aspartame has escalated rapidly, and it is now finding its way into an alarming array of mainstream foods. The worst examples that I found of this were Aspartame in sausages and rice crackers. It is also now found commonly in yoghurts, snacks, desserts, mints, cordials, juices, instant coffee drinks, vitamins and medicines.

Aspartame was first approved for use in 1981, and controversy has simmered since then about the safety of the additive and the circumstances surrounding its approval in the US. Scientists fiercely debated the safety of Aspartame for 20 years prior to its approval. Despite significant scientific data showing a link to the development of brain tumours in rats, the manufacturers, Searle Laboratory, kept pushing for its approval.

One month after approving the additive for use, US Food and Drug Administration Commissioner Arthur Hull Hayes, resigned from his post and became a senior consultant for the public-relations firm that managed Searle's account for Aspartame.

Aspartame is considered by some to be the most dangerous substance on the market that is added to foods. It accounts for over 75% of the adverse reactions reported to the US Food and Drug Administration, yet the additive is still widely permitted and no warning labelling is required.

The range of symptoms and ailments attributed to Aspartame in a 1994 Department of Health and Human Services report include:

> Headache, migraines, dizziness, seizures, numbness, rashes, depression, fatigue, irritability, tachycardia, insomnia, vision problems, hearing loss, heart palpitations, breathing difficulties, slurred speech, tinnitus, vertigo, memory loss and joint pain.

Aspartame is an excitotoxin, just like MSG. Excessive exposure to Aspartame can cause damage to the brain cells and, as with MSG, children and infants (including foetuses) are most at risk because of the undeveloped blood–brain barrier. *For this reason pregnant women should avoid Aspartame, and it should not be given to children at all.*

Aspartame is a compound made up of 50% phenylalanine. Phenylalanine is an amino acid normally found in the brain. People with the genetic disorder called phenylketonuria (PKU) cannot metabolise phenylalanine, and over-exposure can lead to serious complications, even death. For this reason, it's recommended that people with PKU don't consume Aspartame and a warning to this effect is often carried by products, such as diet drinks, containing Aspartame.

However, even people who don't have PKU can develop excessive levels of phenylalanine in the brain after excessive consumption of Aspartame. Excess phenylalanine can cause the levels of serotonin in the brain to decrease, which may lead to emotional disorders such as depression.

Anecdotal evidence exists of people drinking six to eight cans of diet drink daily and experiencing a range of adverse symptoms including mood swings, rages, depression and headaches. These dramatically improved or vanished when Aspartame was removed from their diets.

Aspartame is also linked to brain cancer. It has been shown experimentally to cause brain tumours in rats. In fact, a two-year study by the manufacturer even confirmed this result, yet it was still approved for use!

More recently, scientists from the Ramizzini Institute for Cancer Research in Italy published alarming results from a comprehensive study completed in 2005. This study confirmed that Aspartame caused lymphomas and leukaemia in female animals fed Aspartame *in doses very close to the acceptable daily intake set for humans*. Some of the animals in this study also developed brain tumours.

In 2012 yet another study rang alarm bells about the consumption of aspartame. This study was conducted by a Harvard University teaching facility and published in the American Journal of Nutrition. The study was the longest ever human study undertaken, spanning 22 years. The study evaluated the link between aspartame intake and cancer and found a clear association between aspartame consumption and non–Hodgkins lymphoma and leukemia.

Of great concern also is a possible threat to the health of unborn babies according to a Norwegian study published in August 2012 in the American Journal of Clinical Nutrition. This study of more than 60 000 pregnant women found that those who drank more than one artificially sweetened soda drink a day, were 25 % more likely to give birth prematurely than those who avoided artificially sweetened drinks.

Despite this study there is no move by FSANZ to review or limit the use of Aspartame in Australian foods and, in fact, the use of Aspartame is becoming more and more widespread. It is estimated now that 1 in every 15 people are regular consumers of Aspartame, and many of these are children. As we face a future with half of all Australian kids overweight or obese, more parents are likely to choose "diet" products for their children, and this proportion is going to rise. It is very concerning to think about what the long term effect of regular Aspartame consumption might be in this generation of kids.

It is interesting to note that the incidence of brain cancer in the US, Australia and many other countries has increased substantially since 1981. This coincides with the introduction of Aspartame. It also coincides with the advent of mobile phones and, no doubt, many other coincidences. Still, many researchers aren't surprised at this statistic, given the proven ability of Aspartame to cause brain tumours in animals.

9.5   Other artificial sweeteners

Intense sweeteners are food additives that have a relative sweetness many times that of sugar which means they can be used in much smaller amounts. They are added to foods to replace the sweetness normally provided by sugars without contributing significantly to available energy. This means they offer an enticing appeal to consumers as a means to control kilojoule or carbohydrate intake.

A number of intense sweeteners are approved for use in Australia and New Zealand. These are alitame, acesulfame potassium (Ace K), aspartame, advantame, cyclamate, neotame, saccharin, sucralose, steviol glycosides and thaumatin. However, they often appear on product labels as more appealing sounding brand names such as Nutrasweet, Equal, Spenda or Sweet and Low.

- Saccharin is known to cause cancer in lab animals and is classified as a weak human carcinogen.

- Acesulphame Potassium likewise has been shown to promote tumour growth in laboratory animals, and a large question mark hangs over the safety of its long-term use in humans.

> • Sucralose has been recently added to the Australian Food Standards. There is abundant concern about the safety of this sweetener, and a need for more investigation into its long term use and its effects in humans.
>
> • Cyclamates are regarded as potential carcinogens and have previously been banned from use in foods in the USA and UK due to studies demonstrating links to bladder cancer, but they are still allowed in a wide range of foods and beverages in Australia. Animal studies in existence from the 1970's confirm that cyclamate toxicity results mainly from the action of a breakdown compound, cyclohexylamine, which has been shown to cause testicular atrophy and adverse cardiovascular effects in animal studies. Most concerning is a 2004 FSANZ report which showed that Australian children aged 2 – 11 were exceeding the maximum daily intake of this additive, primarily through consumption of sugar free drinks and juices.

With the growing consumer concern and aversion to taking many of the more common artificial sweeteners, a new breed of "natural" artificial sweeteners has emerged in our food supply. These additives are known as *polyols* and include Sorbitol 420, Mannitol 421, Isomalt 953, Maltitol 965, Lactitol 966, Xylitol 967, Erythritol 968 and Polydextrose 1200.

As with many of the newer additives, there is conflicting information and doubt about the long term safety of these substances. All of these sugar free sweeteners are known to cause gastric upsets and diarrhoea in large doses, and many consumers have reported these symptoms as an adverse side effect of even moderate consumption. *Xylitol* is widely used and promoted as a good choice for diabetics in particular, but some caution is advised as earlier studies did cite a link to cancer. More recent studies have countered these findings, but it may well be sensible to avoid consuming these substances on a regular basis.

Neotame and Advantame are two of the newer artificial sweeteners which are appearing in Australian foods. Both these additives have been developed in response to the ever increasing global consumer aversion to the use of aspartame. However, both these sweeteners are just more intense versions of aspartame, with slightly different chemical structures and with just as many serious concerns surrounding their long term safety. Like aspartame, both neotame and advantame act as excitotoxins once digested and are best avoided. They should definitely not be seen as a safer alternative to the use of aspartame. Neotame was approved for use in Australian in 2001 and Advantame was approved by FSANZ in 2011. Both are found most commonly in beverages and also in some dairy and confectionary products. Neotame is additive number 961 but there is currently no international additive number for Advantame, so it is listed by its name only in the ingredients panel. The safety assessment data available for both of these additives by way of animal or human studies is very thin on the ground. However, some of the animal studies which have been done showed concerning results in relation to endocrine effects and maternal toxicity at high doses.

Of all the sweetener additives available there is one which appears to be the best choice for those people who wish to avoid natural sugars and sweeteners, and that is an additive known as Steviol glycosides.(960). Steviol glycosides are mixtures of steviol glycosides extracted from the leaves of the Stevia plant, a native of Paraguay, which has been used as a natural sweetener in South American countries for centuries. It has also been used in Japan and China as an approved sweetening additive since the 1970's, without any documented ill effects.

Stevia can be found in health food stores in liquid form which is the least processed way of consuming this sweetener. It is intensely sweet, 300 times sweeter than sugar, so a little bit goes a long way. As a result of FSANZ approval in 2008, a full range of stevia based table top sweeteners are now available in supermarkets. These products in tablet, powder and liquid forms are made from steviol glycosides (extracts from the plant) combined with bulking and filling agents, so they are a much more processed form of the sweetener. If you choose to use Stevia, the pure liquid drops would be the most natural form to choose. Be wary of preservatives added to the powder, pill and some drop forms of this product.

9.6 Nitrates and nitrites

Sodium nitrate (250) and sodium nitrite (251) are salt-like chemicals found commonly in processed and cured meats including ham, polony, bacon and frankfurters. They are added to preserve the meats and to add colour and flavour. Their role as a preservative is important as it's the presence of nitrates or nitrites that prevents the bacteria that causes botulism. However, these additives are *widely considered to be toxic and carcinogenic in humans.*

Nitrites are capable of entering the bloodstream and changing the nature of the red blood cells responsible for oxygen transport. When the blood's ability to carry oxygen is impaired, this can lead to a condition known as *methemoglobinemia,* which can result in dizziness, laboured breathing and even death from asphyxiation if nitrite exposure is prolonged. Infants are especially more susceptible to this condition and as such *nitrites aren't permitted in foods intended for infants and young children.*

Nitrites and nitrates are known to react with substances in meats called amines to form compounds known as *nitrosoamines,* which are hazardous poisons and definite animal and human carcinogens. The continued use therefore of nitrate and nitrite preservative in meat products which we eat is a cause for concern for us all. Australians as a population eat a huge amount of processed meats, which means we eat and feed our families a huge amount of nitrate and nitrite preservatives every year. We also have one of the highest rates of bowel cancer in the world and the number of Australians developing bowel cancer is increasing at an alarming rate. The statistics also tell us that Australians are developing bowel cancer at a younger age than has ever been encountered before. It is well established, however, that the single biggest factor influencing bowel cancer rates in developed countries such as ours is our *over consumption of red and processed meats,* especially those containing nitrate and nitrate preservatives.

Official recommendations from the World Cancer Research Fund are to eat no more than 500gm of red meat per week and to avoid completely all processed meats such as ham, polony, hotdogs and salami which are preserved with nitrate chemicals. Naturally preserved nitrate free products including ham, bacon and sausages are however becoming more and more readily available and these are good choices to include in your diet in moderation if you like to eat these types of meats.

Some researchers are very definitive about the risk posed especially to children from the continued consumption of processed meats which have become such common staples in the average Australian child's diet. In his book *Unreasonable Risk,* Dr Samuel Epstein, Chairman of the Cancer Prevention Coalition, provides this excerpt from the Dirty Dozen, a 1995 survey of carcinogens in 12 common consumer products:

Beef frankfurters

Children eating up to about a dozen each month are at an approximately four-fold increased risk of brain cancer and seven-fold increased risk of leukaemia. (This is due to the formation of a nitrosamine carcinogen, by the interaction of nitrate and natural amines in meat.)

Current FSANZ regulations prohibit the use of nitrates and nitrites in foods for infants and young children. However, in effect this only stops the addition of these additives to infant formula and baby food products. What about all the polony, frankfurts and processed meats that most Australian children eat regularly from the age of one and up? Surely, if there's enough evidence of concern to warrant these substances being banned in infants' food, there should be some sort of warning on the labels of other foods containing these substances, so parents can make informed choices about whether or not they want to feed these chemicals to their kids.

Sadly there are more concerns about the effect of nitrates and nitrates in our foods than the clear contributing link to cancer. Nitrates and nitrites are also linked to the ever increasing incidence of dementia and Alzheimer's disease within our population. As with bowel cancer, what is most concerning is not just that the incidence of these diseases are increasing rapidly, but the onset age is becoming younger and younger.

In 2009 a study by researchers at Rhode Island Hospital discovered a substantial link between increased levels of nitrates in our environment and food with increased deaths from diseases such as Alzeihmer's and Parkinson's. The study surmised that as a result of changes to our diets (including our over consumption of processed meats), in combination with an increased environmental exposure (pesticides, fertilisers), people today are exposed to an unprecedented level of nitrosamines which is triggering the increased incidence of these diseases.

Thankfully, it is so easy to limit your exposure to nitrates and nitrites with just a few simple dietary changes. The evidence is clear that this is an important step for us all if we want to avoid colorectal cancers and dementia, but it is especially important that we take steps early to safeguard our childrens' long term health. Consider your own diet and take stock of just how much ham, bacon, processed meats you eat and look at ways of reducing your consumption significantly. If you rely regularly on ham or other processed meats for sandwiches, start to substitute home roasted lamb, chicken or beef, or tinned tuna or salmon instead. Increase your variety by having cheese or egg salad sandwiches, or introduce the habit of cooking a little extra for dinner at night and using your left overs for lunch the next day. With children, get them very used to the fact that processed meat products like ham, polony, kabana and bacon are "sometimes foods" and help them to develop a broader palate by not allowing them have the same sandwich filling every day. It is also possible to source organic nitrate free ham and bacon but these products are more expensive. Many specialty and gourmet butchers supply these products but major supermarkets are also starting to respond to consumer demands and have made these products available also.

In my family we always enjoy an organic nitrate free ham at Christmas time and I have learnt how to cook corned beef the old fashioned way with no nitrates which is a great winter meal. We do still enjoy a ham sandwich from time to time, but I use it as my standby – if the kids are getting lunch from the canteen or we are out and need to buy lunch. Similarly with bacon – I rarely cook bacon at home but if we go out for breakfast we all enjoy an occasional serve of bacon. I don't buy regular ham or bacon as a staple item, but I do buy organic nitrate free ham and bacon when I want to cook with it. Instead of regular ham we eat left over cold roasted meats for lunch and I use the same for home made pizzas and patties. It really is quite easy to dramatically reduce your family's consumption of processed meats with just a little bit of thinking and meal planning, and it really is one of the most important steps you can take to minimise your risk of developing bowel cancer and dementia in later life.

9.7   Artificial colours

Many people are aware of the link between well-known artificial colours and hyperactivity, but far fewer people are aware that many colours widely used in our foods today are proven or suspected carcinogens. As with MSG and Aspartame, the use of colours in our foods seems to be growing all the time, and artificial colours are now found in an amazing array of foods that we eat every day.

Many people who try to avoid the most vibrant artificial colours would be shocked to find out how many colours they are unwittingly consuming every day in seemingly natural, uncoloured foods. Some chocolate biscuits are a good example. Most of us would assume that biscuits such as Tim Tams are made chocolate by the use of cocoa, but in fact that lovely chocolate coating is a mixture of Tartrazine (102), Sunset Yellow (110), Allura Red (129), Brilliant Blue (133), and Caramel (150).

Similarly, many cheese slices these days contain Annatto (160b), Curcumin (100) and Titanium dioxide (171). Fruit juices and juice drinks are another common source of a daily dose of artificial colours including Caramel (150), which is found in many apple drinks, and Sunset Yellow (110) and Tartrazine (102), which are found in many orange-flavoured drinks.

It is this widespread use of colours in our foods that is concerning, especially when the use of colours is purely a manufacturing ploy to enhance the appeal of a product to consumers. Colours in food perform no function other than cosmetic. They are there just to make the food look better to the consumer.

It can be argued that in many cases the colours are used to fool the consumer by making inferior products look more enticing and real. Whatever the reasons, we're now consuming more of these substances in our diets than ever before. Their use is so widespread in processed foods that, in the US, it's estimated that the average daily consumption of artificial colours ranges from *15 to 50 milligrams per person per day*. We can assume that Australian dietary trends would reflect this level of consumption also.

Once again, this is most concerning in relation to children, as it's in children's foods that we see the most obvious and heaviest overuse of artificial colours. The insidious appearance of colours in staple foods such as fruit juice, cheese, margarines and biscuits is alarming, especially when parents trying to limit consumption of colours by their families, may well be unaware that these basic food items contain a wide range of colouring additives.

The health concerns associated with colours are varied. The most well known effect is hyperactivity. This applies mainly to a range of colours known as the Coal Tar and AZO dyes. These include 102, 104, 110, 122, 123, 124, 132, 133, 142, 151 and 155. Over the past 20 years, more than a dozen of these types of additives have been taken off the market following laboratory confirmation that they were toxic or carcinogenic. Many of these additives have not been reviewed in relation to safety for 30 years or more, and, for many, the original safety testing was minimal and inconclusive. In 2007, the European Food Standards Agency initiated a systematic review of some colour additives due to mounting concern over their long term safety and lack of accurate safety data. While this process will take many years to complete, the first additive reviewed under this project, colour Red 2G, was found to be likely carcinogenic and immediately recalled from use.

Abundant concern also exists surrounding the effect of these additives on children, particularly adverse behaviour and learning impacts. A 2003 study published by the respected *Archives of Disease in Childhood,* found that some colour additives can have an adverse effect on all children, not just those prone to hyperactivity or allergies. The results of this study were confirmed in September 2007 in a repeat study commissioned by the UK Food Standards Agency and conducted by the University of Southhampton. The results of the most recent study were published in *The Lancet* and clearly confirmed the wealth of anecdotal experience linking colours and preservatives to adverse behaviour effects in children.

The research was conducted using 3 year olds and 8 – 9 year olds, and, importantly, the findings confirmed again that the additives caused adverse effects within the *general population* and not just those kids with a history of hyperactivity or ADHD. The "significantly adverse effects" observed included tantrums, poor concentration and slow progress at school.

The additives tested in the study were colours Sunset Yellow (110), Tartrazine (102), Carmoisine (122), Ponceau 4R (124), Quinoline Yellow (104), Allura Red (129) and preservative Sodium Benzoate (211). Combinations of these additives are commonly found in childrens' products such as cordials, fruit juices, museli bars, yoghurts, fruit sticks, milk drinks as well as confectionary and soft drink.

In the wake of these findings the UK food Safety Authority introduced a voluntary withdrawal of the 6 colour additives which came into effect in July 2010. In addition, the European Parliament introduced new legislation demanding that explicit warning labels be required for any product which continued to use any of the 6 colour additives after 2010. This legislation is now fully in force across the whole EU. Any product which continues to use any of the 6 colours must display a label stating: ***Warning: Contains food additives that may have an adverse effect on activity and attention.*** Clearly such labelling has resulted in the complete removal of these 6 additives from food products in the EU as no manufacturer wants to have labels such as these attached to their product. The European Food Safety Authority also decreased the acceptable daily intake levels (ADI) for 3 of these colours yet our food regulator again has refused to follow their lead..

In fact, here in Australia, FSANZ, has done absolutely nothing to reduce the use of these chemicals in our foods or to even raise awareness amongst consumers that these colours can cause problems. Following on from the action in Europe in 2007 consumer advocates here joined forces with Additive Alert and launched the Kids First Campaign, calling on our regulator to follow the lead of the UK FSA, and remove these additives from our food or, at the very least, introduce a requirement for warning labels as per the EU parliament action. Despite more than 250 000 Australians petitioning our food regulator, FSANZ refused to take any action at all on these colours aside from issuing a statement that *"parents of hyperactive children may wish to avoid these additives"*.

This completely inadequate response does nothing to assist parents to make sound choices for their kids, and completely misses the central point of the study findings, that these additives have now been shown to be of concern for all children, not just children with hyperactivity problems.

Despite assertions from FSANZ that these colours are not used in many products in Australia, a survey conducted by the Food Intolerance Network found more than 1000 everyday products which continue to use these colours. They are found in obvious sources such as confectionary, cordials, ice cream and jellies, but also in less obvious sources such as muesli bars, fruit juices, muffins, breads, wraps, cakes, rice crackers, tinned fruit, fruit sicks, flavoured milks, asian noodles, cooking sauces, yoghurts and breakfast cereals– all common products that many children are eating on a very regular basis.

Several colours still permitted in Australia have previously been banned in other countries because of their proven links to cancer. These colours include Amaranth (123), Food Green (142), Brilliant Black (151), Carbon Black (153) and Brown HT (155). There are many other colours permitted in Australia that are strongly suspected of being carcinogenic based on animal tests, but are still widely used, mainly in children's foods, with no warnings required on the labels. In 2010 the leading consumer advocacy group in the US, the Centre for Science in the Public Interest (CSPI) released a detailed report titled Food Dyes: A Rainbow of Risks. The report was presented to the US FDA and called for the removal of 7 common food dyes from the food supply, due to scientific evidence that these additives were unsafe. CSPI executive director and report co-author Michael F. Jacobson said the colours had been shown to cause cancer in rats and trigger behavioural problems in children. *"These synthetic chemicals do absolutely nothing to improve the nutritional quality or safety of foods but trigger behaviour problems in children and, possibly, cancer in anybody,"* Mr Jacobson said. However, as at 2017, no action has been taken by the US FDA or our own regulator here to remove these colours from our food supply.

Other "natural" colour additives such as Annatto (160b) are believed to be associated with behaviour and learning impairment, especially in children. This additive is becoming more and more widespread and is commonly found in foods that are coloured white, cream or yellow including cheese and margarine.

Although Annatto is regarded as safe in Australia it is interesting to note that some studies have implicated this additive as a possible trigger in hypersensitivity reactions including urticaria, eczema, angioedma and even anaphylaxis. With the ever increasing incidence of potentially fatal true food allergy in Australia, especially amongst children, this is important for consumers to be aware of, as the use of annatto in our foods is becoming more and more common.

The safety of another "natural" additive Curcumin (100) similarly is still far from assured. Initial safety assessments raised questions about a potential to cause genetic damage and conception risks. High doses are also known to enhance the release of bile from the liver, raising queries about its long term safety for people with gallstones or liver problems. Whilst the research and re assessment wheels grind away slowly, these additives are included in our food supplies, with no warnings required, as more testing is done.

Tartrazine (102) is another insidious colour that is now found in many foods including juices. It is linked to a wide array of health problems including irritability, gastric upsets and sleep disturbances. Breastfeeding mothers have found that eliminating this additive has helped their "colicky" babies sleep better and be less fretful. It is also known to disrupt the body's metabolism of zinc and is implicated as a contributing factor in ADD and ADHD in some children.

One of the main problems in relation to determining the safety or otherwise of these substances lies in the initial testing. Prior to introduction, additives are tested for acute toxicity, but even if laboratory tests show links to cancer or other serious side effects, this doesn't necessarily mean that they will be prohibited. As we have seen, despite clear evidence in animal tests that a substance does cause damage, a lower "safe" level of consumption is determined, and often these additives go on to be included in our foods.

These additives also aren't tested for *neuropsychological* effects such as hyperactivity and subtle behaviour and learning impacts. Also, they are tested in isolation, not in combination, which is how they are actually consumed in our diets.

This is why there's so much conflicting evidence about the safety of many of these substances. As consumers, *we need to remember that just because these additives are currently permitted in our foods, it doesn't guarantee that they are safe.*

When shopping, the best rule of thumb is to avoid any obviously coloured foods, and don't assume that plain coloured foods are necessarily colour free. White ice cream usually contains a couple of colours, and chocolate-flavoured biscuits, ice creams and drinks are often made brown by blending several of the most toxic colour additives.

Be on the look out also for subtle colours such as Caramel and Annatto. These colours are often marketed aggressively using the label *No Artificial Colours*. As we have seen, this in no way means they are actually any better or safer for us.

9.8   Preservatives

Preservatives are a necessary addition to processed foods if we want to have access to products that will remain fresh. Once again, however, the use of preservatives is growing rapidly, and we're now finding more and more preservatives creeping into our staple foods such as bread, fruit juice, margarine and even supposedly fresh meats and fish. For this reason consumers need to be aware of the health impacts associated with the different groups of preservatives.

Unlike colours, most preservatives are generally not linked to cancer, but other serious concerns are held about the long-term cumulative effect of these additives in our diets. Some preservative groups are known to be dangerous to asthmatics, whilst others are known to contribute to behaviour and learning problems, especially in sensitive children. Unlike reactions to colours, which are often dramatic and obvious, reactions to preservatives are often delayed and subtle, and therefore difficult to identify and pinpoint.

Preservatives found to cause problems are described in the following sections.

9.9   Sulphites (220–228)

Sulphites are a group of preservative additives which once were only commonly used in wine production and dried fruit products. Consequently, our traditional consumption of these preservatives has been a very small proportion of our diet. Swing the clock forward through to 2017 and sulphite preservatives are ubiquitous in our foods, in everything from breakfast cereals and muesli bars, baby foods, fruit juices, cordials, fresh fruit and even fresh meat and fresh fish. As a result, Australian consumers, and especially Australian children, are eating more sulphite preservatives in our everyday foods than ever before, and there are very valid concerns about the impacts this shift may be having on our health.

Sulphite preservatives have been shown to trigger asthma attacks in sufferers. The sulphur dioxide gas (a major irritant to asthmatics) contained in sulphites is released and inhaled when food is ingested. For this reason, the World Health Organisation recommends that anyone susceptible to asthma should avoid food and drinks containing sulphites, and this advice is particularly important for children with asthma.

These additives are also of wider concern as 220 is a suspected mutagen and possible teratogen, and is linked to a variety of ill effects in animal studies including gastric irritation and liver toxicity. Worldwide, as the consumption of sulphites increases, evidence of much broader adverse effects is also becoming more apparent. Sulphites have been implicated in allergic and anaphylactic type reactions as well as nausea, sinus irritation, headaches, migraine, rashes and behavioural impacts, so many people, not just asthmatics, may wish to avoid or limit their consumption of sulphites.

Whilst sulphite preservatives in packaged foods do need to be labelled, it can be difficult to avoid them in unpackaged foods like fresh meat. Once an unheard of practice in Australian meat retailers, it is now common practice for meat vendors to sprinkle sodium metabisulphite powder on mince and meat products to keep the produce looking red and fresh. This is an illegal practice in Australia, but a 2005 survey by Choice magazine found that almost 50% of butchers were adding illegal sulphites to their meat, and the practice continues to be widespread today. Fresh mince is the most commonly contaminated product. The sulphites wont be listed on the label (because its illegal) but you can check your meat easily yourself just by a simple observation experiment.

Fresh meat is not supposed to remain intensely red in colour after it has been sliced and exposed to the air. The retailers are adding the sulphites to the meat to retain the red colour, to make the meat look fresher and more appealing. In its natural state, all meat will lose its bright red colour and move to a duller brown/ pink as the surface of the meat reacts with oxygen in the air. This is normal and does not mean the meat is off or old, but the use of sulphites in meat has become so common practice that most of us can not even remember what real meat is meant to look like! The retailers love to use the sulphite powder on our meat because it makes us think the meat is fresher and enables them to keep older produce which may not sell, looking fresh and appealing. So switch your eyes on next time you buy meat. If the mince is really red on the outside but a dull brown/ pink colour on the inside then you know the meat has been "sulphited". Similarly, if you buy mince and take it home and put in the fridge, after a day or 2 the surface of the meat should dull in colour – if it doesn't, again, you know you have got some sneaky sulphites added to your meat.

In August 2005 FSANZ released the results from their 21st Total Diet Study into the consumption of sulphites, benzoates and sorbates. This study revealed that a significant proportion of the population takes in more than the Acceptable Daily Intake

(ADI) of sulphites and benzoates, particularly for children ages 2-5 years who, according to the report, may be taking in up to four times the sulphite ADI. Since these figures are based on food consumption in 1995, well before the explosion of dried fruit based snacks for kids, it is extremely likely that these findings seriously underestimate actual consumption, especially by children.

The reality is that today's children especially are eating an unprecedented level of sulphite preservatives in everyday food. The fact that we in Australia also have one of the highest childhood asthma rates in the world should also give us pause for thought that perhaps there may be a connection. The evidence is very clear that very small amounts of sulphite preservatives can be very troublesome to adults and children who are susceptible to asthma. So, if you or your children are affected by asthma, then it may well be a very wise move to actively take steps to minimise your sulphite consumption as much as you can. This may mean changing your breakfast cereal and fruit juice and steering away from packaged muesli bars and dried fruit snacks, but this is a whole lot easier and safer than ending up in hospital with an asthma attack after eating a few dried apricots.

It can be a real eye opener for many people to take stock of just how many sulphites are being consumed on a daily basis, especially hidden in so called "healthy" food options. For anyone with asthma or respiratory type symptoms, an elimination of sulphites could be a really smart and easy experiment to undertake. Similarly, for adults and children with skin disorders or recurrent sinus problems, eliminating sulphites and other problem additives has been shown to help correct a multitude of common chronic health complaints. Look out for breakfast cereal and museli bar type products, anything with dried fruit, fruit juices, cordials, wine and alcoholic drinks, fresh mince and fresh seafood, especially prawns which often have sulphite powder routinely and liberally sprinkled over them on the boats. Finally, check your fresh fruit. With so much fruit from all over the world being available all year round, some products such as grapes are often routinely sprayed with sulphites to help preserve their freshness. If buying fruit out of season which is not local, it always pays to check as sulphites on fresh produce are often not labelled.

9.10 Propionates (280–283)

Just like their sulphite preservative cousins, propionate preservatives were rarely used in Australian foods a generation ago, and were certainly not found in everyday staples like bread. In 2017 however, these preservatives are used prolifically in most bread and bakery products and are also starting to appear in other everyday healthy food items such as fruit juices, cheese and dried fruit products.

Propionates are associated with an array of adverse health problems including behaviour and learning problems, lethargy, gastro-intestinal problems, migraines, irritability, depression, sleep disturbances and growing pains. They are also implicated in causing the same symptoms and great distress in babies who are exposed through breast milk.

Calcium propionate (282) is appearing more and more commonly in our foods, not just in fresh bread products. All mainstream breadcrumb products contain this additive. So, to avoid it, you need to either make your own breadcrumbs or look for organic varieties. It is also in many prepared frozen foods such as some fish fingers and many products coated with or containing breadcrumbs. Many frozen sausage rolls contain bread crumbs in the mix. These will contain 282, but it will likely not be declared on the label. If an ingredient label lists breadcrumbs but the breakdown of the breadcrumbs isn't provided, you would need to ring and check to find out if 282 is in the product.

Calcium propionate is banned in the UK because it is known to cause skin rashes in bakery workers. An Australian study conducted in the Northern Territory confirmed that consumption of this additive can adversely affect children's behaviour. The results of this study were published in the Journal of Paediatrics and Child Health in 2002, and confirm that propionates appear to have a dramatic effect on many children in relation to behaviour, attention, disposition and general happiness.

There is also a wealth of anecdotal evidence from mothers linking this additive to sleeping and gastrointestinal problems in young babies, with many women reporting that colicky, restless babies improved significantly when this additive is removed from the mother's diet.

Once again, it is the effect on this generation of children that is really of most concern. Australian children eat a lot of bread and bread products and most would be eating propionate preservatives every day, often numerous doses. To make matters worse, Australia also has one of the highest permitted levels in the world of propionate preservatives allowed in foods. Like all additives, these preservatives were not tested before approval for their effects on children's behaviour, concentration and learning ability. Since that time though, it has become clear that these preservatives do in fact have very definite adverse impacts on these areas, and high does are known to be neurotoxic. In 2012 Canadian researchers demonstrated that excess levels of propionic acid in the diet could accumulate in cells and cause adverse effects on brain development and function, leading to a hypothesis that propionates may be implicated in some way in the increasing rates of autism.

Clearly there is still so much we do not know about the effect of additives such as these in our foods, especially the long term effects on our children, so it make very good sense to avoid these inconspicuous additives as much as you can.

As consumer awareness and avoidance of additives such as calcium propionate increases, however, the manufacturers often respond by finding new ways of hiding these additives in our foods. Due to consumer backlash about the use of 282 in so many bread products, a new wave of *"282 free"* products have become available on our shelves. The main culprits are bread and bread products such as wraps in which he manufacturers have started using ingredients such as whey, dextrose or wheat that has been cultured with propionic bacteria to create a " natural" form of propionate preservative. Under the labelling laws in place this subtle change in manufacturing process means that the end product still contains propionates in significant levels, but the manufacturers are not required to list propionates on their labels as a preservative. This is not just wrong, its also dangerous, especially for those people including children, who have asthma triggered by propionates or whose health is otherwise adversely affected by propionates.

9.11 Benzoates (210–213)

Benzoates are found in soft drinks and particularly cordials. They also are considered dangerous for asthmatics and people sensitive to Aspirin (salicylates). They are also linked more widely to a range of adverse effects including hyperactivity, eye and skin irritation, and gastric burning. Sodium benzoate (211) is associated with liver, kidney and neurotoxic effects and is also regarded as a possible teratogen.

Benzoates are quickly gaining a reputation as one of the worst additives in relation to provoking behaviour and learning problems in children. Research published in 2004 in the peer review journal *Archives of Disease in Childhood* confirmed that benzoate preservatives have a negative effect on children's behaviour across the board, not just those prone to hyperactivity or allergies. The findings of this report detailed that all the 3-year-olds involved in the study reacted negatively to benzoates, but some were more sensitive than others, reacting at a lower dose. This confirmed that reactions to these preservatives are *dose related and cumulative*, making it extremely difficult for people to make the connection between health or behaviour problems and benzoate consumption until the additives are removed from the diet completely and then retested.

Children today are consuming more benzoate preservatives than ever before. Benzoates are now being used by manufacturers more and more in drinks other than soft drinks and cordials. They are now found commonly in fruit juices, sports drinks and many water substitutes which are marketed directly at children and school canteens, meaning that more and more children are consuming these additives on a regularly or daily basis in drinks which are perceived by the children and parents as "healthy" choices.

Benzoates have also been linked more recently to another seriously worrying side effect that is of concern to us all, not just asthmatics or children. In 2006 it was revealed that authorities in the USA and UK had found disturbing levels of cancer causing *benzene* residue in many popular brands of soft drink. Following on from the alarming findings overseas, FSANZ conducted some testing of drinks in Australia. Their report confirmed that of the 68 samples tested, 38 had benzene levels from 1-40 ppb, meaning that **more than half** the drinks tested had benzene levels well above the Australian guidelines for drinking water of 1ppb.

Benzene is a nasty chemical linked to cancers, particularly leukaemia. It can form in soft drinks that contain two specific ingredients: Vitamin C (ascorbic acid), and either sodium benzoate or potassium benzoate. Researchers speculate that benzoates can break down in the presence of heat or light into benzene. Regardless of why it is happening, benzene is not something that any of us should be drinking on a regular basis, especially not our children.

In May 2007 yet another red flag emerged in relation to the safety of benzoate preservatives. Research from the University of Sheffield was released claiming that laboratory studies could demonstrate that sodium benzoate could cause serious cell damage at the DNA level. Study head, Professor Peter Piper, released the worrying discovery that benzoates and sorbates are capable of causing extensive damage to an important area of DNA in the power station of cells known as the mitochondria. Speaking in Australia in November 2007 at the *Food Industry and Labelling Conference*, Professor Piper provided the international keynote address on his findings. He stressed that these new results must be investigated further as a matter of priority, as the original safety studies completed on both benzoates and sorbates would not have been able to detect these types of changes due to the limitations of technology at the time.

There is no need to expose yourself or your family to these chemicals in your diet. There are plenty of safe preservatives available which can be used instead of benzoates and sorbates, and there are plenty of good choices on offer in the shops. So have a good look at your fruit juices, cordials and sports drinks and steer clear of products containing benzoates wherever possible.

9.12 Dried fruit and fresh fruit

Most conventional dried fruit available in the supermarket today is preserved by the use of sulphur dioxide (220) or potassium sorbate (202). As has been discussed earlier, sulphite preservatives have a raft of concerns associated with their regular consumption, and sorbates similarly are associated with asthma, behavioural problems and other adverse effects. Sorbates are commonly found in dried fruit products, as well as bread products (as an alternative to the more well known calcium propionate), and also are becoming more and more common in dairy products such as cream or cottage cheese and fruit juices.

Dried apricots and dried apples are both readily available in organic form (even major supermarkets now have in-house organic ranges) so it is easy to source non preserved options. The only difference will be in the appearance of the fruit. The sulphite preservatives help to retain the colour of the apricots in particular – non preserved organic apricots will be brown not orange in colour, but they taste exactly the same. Thankfully sultanas and dates usually are not treated with preservatives, but be aware that some sultana products are often covered with vegetable oil, which may have an unlisted antioxidant present. Again, sourcing organic sultanas is the easiest option here, or look for natural sultanas which do not have vegetable oil listed as an ingredient.

Fresh fruit, incredibly, is fast becoming a new source of concern when it comes to avoiding additives. Due primarily to changes in our food supply, we have experienced a shift from sourcing fresh and locally grown fruit and vegetables to a mass produced system which means that often the fruit and vegetables we find in our local store have come from the other side of the world and may be many months old in some cases. In order to be able to do this, the fruit and vegetable industry rely on numerous additives and packing techniques to keep the produce "fresh".

Grapes are routinely available now all year round which means that they often originate from the other side of the world. To keep them "fresh", sulphur dioxide is used to prevent mould growth but this is rarely disclosed at point of sale.

According to *Choice* magazine (Nov 2010) apples found in our supermarkets could be up to 1 year old, but are preserved to look fresh by being harvested unripe, kept in cold storage and treated with 1-methylcyclopropene, a plant growth and ripening regulation chemical, but again this information is not disclosed to us at point of sale. The same chemical is routinely used on other fruits and vegetables including avocados, kiwifruit, plums pears and many others.

Irradiation of our food is another emerging trend which most consumers are unaware of. It is already permissible in Australia for some tropical fruits, berries, tomatoes and capsicums to be irradiated prior to sale to protect against moulds, bacteria and pests. However, as of 2017, FSANZ is considering expanding the scope of the current food code permissions to enable producers to irradiate a much wider range of fruit and vegetable produce including apples, melons, stone fruit, zuchinni and squash. Whilst the official advice regarding food irradiation is that is considered a safe process which does not impact human health, this is by no way a definitive conclusion, and many consumers and advocacy groups worldwide would much prefer that their food was not deliberately exposed to radiation before they eat it.

And it gets worse. In 2012 FSANZ approved the use of a novel processing aid known as Listex P100, which is permitted to be added to ready to eat non liquid foods such as freshly prepared salad, processed meats, seafood and cheeses. This additive is a *bacteriophage*. It is in fact an *engineered group of viruses* which is capable of destroying the toxic bacteria know as Listeria, often found in cold, prepacked ready to eat foods such as the ones listed above. Listeria in our foods was once a rare thing and mainly pregnant women were careful to avoid possible sources such as soft cheeses and pate, as it can have fatal consequence for the unborn child. In recent years though the rate of Listeria infection has increased, particularly amongst the elderly, and the sources of Listeria contamination have expanded from soft cheese and pate, to processed meats, seafood, and prepacked, salads and salad leaves. The more a product is handled prior to point of sale, the higher the chance of Listeria contamination, so it is understandable that our increased consumption of prepacked salads has led to an increase in Listeria, although ironic that our attempts to eat a healthy food could be exposing us to illness! Once again, thanks to FSANZ, the presence of Listex P100 is not declared on the label, but if you buy prepacked salads in particular, it is very likely that the produce will have been treated. In 2016 FSANZ also quietly approved the introduction of another engineered bacteriophage patented as Salmonelex, which is now being applied direct to our fresh meat, seafood and poultry as a salmonella preventative measure. FSANZ has classified its use as a processing aid so it also is not required to be declared on the label.

One final watch out for with dried fruit, fresh fruit and nuts is the continued use of additives such as propylene glycol (1520) which is used to help retain moisture. Propylene glycol is extremely toxic in high doses and has been shown to be a neurotoxin linked to central nervous system depression. It is not something which should be in our foods, even in small amounts, so do check your labels for this additive in particular and search for a better alternative if you can.

9.13 Antioxidants

Antioxidants are found widely in our foods in just about all products that contain oil or fat in any form. As we have seen previously, in many cases these additives aren't listed on the labels because they are present in amounts of less than 5% of an ingredient. Unfortunately, their use is so widespread that all small percentages of hidden antioxidants do add up. For many people, this can cause serious adverse health effects.

The worst aspect of the use of suspect antioxidants in our foods is that there are many safe alternatives that could be used by manufacturers, but these are more expensive and so are overlooked in favour of cheaper substances.

Antioxidants 300–309 are all safe and effective, and manufacturers using these antioxidants are to be applauded. However antioxidants 310–312 and 319–321 are *extremely questionable* and should be avoided wherever possible. Apart from their individual toxic characteristics these antioxidants are also suspected of being dangerous to asthmatics.

9.14 Propyl, octyl and dodecyl-gallate (310–312)

These substances are highly irritant to asthmatics and are all prohibited in foods for infants and young children, yet they are commonly found in many foods that children eat on a regular basis. They are known to cause skin irritations and gastric upsets and should also be avoided by those people sensitive to aspirin or salicylates. They are suspected carcinogens and 312 caused death in animal tests. They should all be avoided and especially not given to children or consumed by pregnant and breastfeeding women.

9.15 Tert-butylhydroquinone or TBHQ (319)

This additive is found most often in snack foods and some savoury biscuits as an additive in the oil and is often not labelled. A dose of 5 grams is known to be fatal to an adult, but manufacturers aren't required to list how much of the additive is present in the food. It is a suspected carcinogen and is linked to birth defects. Ingestion can cause nausea, vomiting, delirium and collapse. It should be avoided in particular by infants, young children and pregnant or breastfeeding women.

9.16 Butylated hydroxyanisole or BHA (320)

This is probably the most common of the suspect antioxidants that most people should avoid. It is found widely in sweet and savoury biscuits, margarine, peanut butter, ice-cream cones, frozen foods and mayonnaise, *even though it's prohibited in foods intended for infants and young children.*

It is of particular concern because it accumulates in the body fat, so residual levels increase over time as more and more is consumed. It is a known animal carcinogen and produces detrimental reproductive effects in animal tests. It is a suspected human carcinogen and acts as a xeno-oestrogen (a substance that mimics the effects of oestrogen) stimulating the growth of breast cells in laboratory cultures. Apart from its strong links to cancer, it should be avoided, especially by children, because of its ability to disrupt the body's hormone balance in this way.
Recent research in New Zealand is also looking into a possible link between BHA and asthma, in particular the use of this additive in dairy produce such as margarines.

Because of the cumulative effect of BHA, it's worthwhile finding out for sure what you're eating and what you're feeding to your kids.

9.17 Butylated hydroxytoluene or BHT (321)

In experimental animals, BHT has proven to be a teratogen and carcinogen and produces adverse effects on reproductive organs. In rat experiments the number of births decreased as the dose of BHT increased, and it induced benign and malignant growths in the livers. It is strongly suspected of being a human teratogen also. Once again because of such serious health impacts and the possibility that it may contribute to birth defects, it's an additive to be avoided wherever possible, *especially by children and pregnant and breastfeeding women.*

9.18 Avoiding the nasty antioxidants - can it be done?

The simple answer is yes, and its not that hard. Thankfully, there are many products available which are opting to avoid the unsafe antioxidants and switch to the safer alternatives, and these are the products we definitely want to support. We also want to send a strong message to those other manufacturers that we, as consumers, don't want to eat toxic substances in our foods and we simply won't buy their products. Since Additive Alert was first published in 2004 there has been a very encouraging shift in the food manufacturing industry away from using cheaper synthetic antioxidants in favour of the safer options, and this has been driven entirely by Australian consumers choosing the safer products at the checkout.

Unfortunately however, because of the 5% labelling loophole, there are still many products on our supermarket shelves which contain undeclared antioxidants. Any product that has oils or fats listed in their ingredient list probably also has an antioxidant to stop the oil from going off. Frozen pastry products, frozen meals, cooking sauces and biscuits, crackers and chips all commonly do not have their antioxidants listed. So, to avoid eating antioxidants that you really don't want to consume, first, read your labels and look for the safer ones, and, then, if you see oils or fats on the ingredients list but no antioxidant declared, make a phone call and ask if an antioxidant is hiding there. If they are using a suspect one, take the opportunity then and there to tell them that you won't be buying their product – this type of feedback is very powerful and really does effect change.

Chapter 10: So what's left?

10.1 Decision time

Having read this far, you're probably either feeling really motivated to reduce your intake of certain additives or else you're feeling overwhelmed and a bit depressed about what this new knowledge might mean to your eating habits.

Well don't despair — it's really not that hard to make a few very simple changes to your eating habits that will greatly reduce your exposure to harmful additives and improve your health.

The first thing you need to do is to decide which additives you want to avoid. This will depend upon your own health and circumstances, but a summary list of the most concerning additives is provided in *Appendix 1* on page 101 for your reference. For example, if asthma isn't a problem in your family then you may not be too concerned about sulphites and some preservatives. Alternately, you may decide that you want to eliminate all additives with *any* known adverse health effects from your diet.

Even if you don't have any specific health concerns at the moment, it makes sense for each of us to make some informed decisions about the food we eat and feed our families. As we have seen previously, the amount of additives we're all consuming every day has grown exponentially over the past 50 years.

A recent study in the UK estimated that by age 18, most children would have consumed half their body weight in food additives.

Knowing what we now know about the potential toxicity of many of these additives, this has to be concerning. Making a decision to reduce your family's intake of all suspect additives may not have an immediately obvious benefit, but it can only do your family's health good to eat less additives, especially those with question marks surrounding their long term safety.

The very good news is that choosing low-additive foods doesn't mean boring foods. In the main, there are better low-additive choices across all the main product ranges, so in many cases you can still eat the same sort of food, just a different brand. For a clear example of how you can shop smarter and pick the best brands to drastically reduce your additive intake, have a look at the *Additive Consumption Comparison table* on Page 92.

Remember though, that junk is still junk, and highly processed and refined snack foods should not feature prominently in a good, healthy-eating plan anyway. We should be trying to eat less processed and packaged food and more fresh food. In this way, you'll avoid a great number of unnecessary additives in your diet.

Deciding to go low additive doesn't mean that another barbecue-flavoured corn chip or chocolate biscuit will never pass your lips. What this does mean is that you'll choose to eat these foods much less frequently than before, and when you do eat them, you'll be well aware of what you're doing and what's in the food you're eating.

10.2 Changing the habits of a lifetime

The guiding principle in making long-term dietary change is to take it slowly. Don't feel as if you have to empty out your pantry and fridge and restock everything from scratch. If you try to do this, you'll probably get overwhelmed and give up, and it will cost you a fortune.

Approach the change *gradually*, and you'll be much more likely to make changes that you'll stick to and which will become your normal eating habits within a very short time.

Focus on becoming aware of what you're eating now, identify the most important changes to make, and change your product choices accordingly, bit by bit.

> How to start changing the habits of a lifetime
>
> - Start with your staples like bread, margarine, cereals, biscuits, juice, canned foods, lunchmeats and fillings, and cooking sauces.
>
> - Have a quick look at the labels of the brands you buy and see if they contain the things you now know you want to avoid.
>
> - If they do, pick one item at a time, then next time you need to restock that item, allow a little extra time to read the labels of just that one product and find a better choice.

It may take a few weeks, but it's better to do it bit by bit than to take on too much and give up. By making the changes gradually, as you need to restock items, you'll find that you very quickly end up with better choices in your house, at the very least for the staple foods you eat every day.

Once you have sorted out your staple grocery choices, do the same with the other products you buy every week. It may seem like a big task at first, but if you approach it systematically like this, it will only be a few weeks until you have found better brands for most things, and you'll have eliminated a huge amount of unnecessary, possibly dangerous additives from your everyday diet.

For example, for many Australians, *Arnott's Tim Tams* are the go to choice when it comes to a decadent chocolate biscuit. How many people realize, however, that there is not a lot of real chocolate in these biscuits? Instead, Arnott's use a variety of combinations of artificial colours such as Allura Red, Tartrazine and Brilliant Blue to create the illusion of a decadent chocolate biscuit! Paradoxically though, other Arnott's chocolate biscuit products, such as *Caramel Crowns*, do not contain any artificial colours at all. Simply by swapping one biscuit for another, it is that easy to avoid a whole host of undesirable additives. Lets be clear though - in no way am I suggesting that *Arnotts Caramel*

Crown is a healthier choice! A chocolate biscuit is a chocolate biscuit full of unhealthy fats and sugar, but, if you are going to eat a chocolate biscuit, at least pick one made from real food ingredients without the unnecessary chemical cocktail!

Similarly, instead of choosing a butter spread such as *Devondale Extra Soft* which contains sorbate preservatives and artificial flavours, you could swap to *Mainland Butter Soft* which contains just milk, cream and salt. Again, a simple choice which eliminates questionable additives from your everyday diet.

It really is all a matter of choice and, with the information you know have, it's easy to incorporate the safer choices into your daily eating habits. In addition to cutting out harmful additives, a lot of additive conscious shoppers also find that by paying attention to which additives are in foods, they also start to pay greater attention to the actual nutrition conferred in the foods they eat. Often they end up choosing better quality foods with less additives, less salt, less sugar, less processing and better all round nutrition, a flow on effect which can only be seen as beneficial in the long term.

Chapter 11: Healthier low-additive eating guidelines

11.1 Introduction

We all know that we should be eating more fruit and vegetables and that most of us don't eat enough whole foods. With the current obesity crisis facing Australia, as in most western countries, governments and health officials are trying hard to educate us all about better eating to try to turn around the worrying trend towards obesity, especially amongst our children. However being educated about what we should eat and translating that into practice are two entirely different matters.

As a nation, we don't eat our two fruit and five vegetables every day, and we eat far too much processed food. We eat too much salt and sugar and nowhere near enough fibre. The changes in our dietary habits over the past 50 years reflect the ever increasing pace of our lives, and therein lies a big problem when it comes to additives

Busy lives mean less time. It means people want convenient food that looks good, tastes good, is quick to cook and lasts a long time. The cost of such convenience is a staggering blow to our overall health and nutrition and a huge increase in the consumption of additives every day.

Here are some basic shopping and eating principles that are simple to adopt but which can make a big difference to your overall health and wellbeing. In the main, these changes won't cost you anything, but they may make a huge difference to your health in the long run. All you need is a desire to eat better and the dedication to use the information you now have to your best advantage.

11.2 Increase your fruit and vegetable consumption

We all should eat at least two fruit and five vegetables a day but how many of us do? This is one thing you really should work on. Even if you can't get up to two and five, at least aim to improve by 50% whatever you manage now.

Try to get one fruit in with your breakfast (and don't skip breakfast!) and another in as a snack throughout the day. Eating five vegetables is easy to achieve if you just plan your meals. Try to get some salad in with your lunch and at least three sorts of vegies on your plate for the evening meal. A lot of us are very conditioned to eating carbohydrate heavy breakfasts such as cereal or toast every single day – we tend to be creatures of habit. These standard breakfast options are quick, easy and tasty and, in the past, we have been warned not to eat too many eggs for fear of cholesterol problems. However, with the latest science confirming that eggs are not an enemy to our health, we can enjoy more egg and protein based breakfasts without worry.

Try to vary your breakfasts and enjoy a cooked breakfast several days a week, and take the opportunity to add in some vegies to boost your intake. Cooked tomatoes, spinach and mushrooms are all great quick, easy and tasty additions to an omelette. Just a simple change such as this can greatly boost your vegetable intake every week. Also, don't be scared of leftovers for breakfast. Soups, stews and casseroles which contain meat and vegies are all delicious choices for breakfast, served with or without a slice of toast, which can help to up your average vegetable intake. At lastly, don't forget the baked beans. Although carbohydrate heavy, beans are full of fibre and good nutrition and make a tasty breakfast, especially in winter. Jazz them up a with a little bit of cooked tomato, grated zuchinni, carrot and mushrooms and you have a very sustaining meal option, and an extra serve or two of vegetables in your day.

Be creative with kids, and hide them if you have to. (The vegies, not the kids!) Grate some zucchini and carrot inside an omelette. Add some mashed, cooked vegies to sausage rolls. Add veggies to your pizza toppings, and only allow treat foods like tinned spaghetti if it has some vegies mixed in with it. Pasta is a perennial favourite with children and this is the easiest way in adding in extra vegies that will not be met with sustained resistance. Blended soups are a good option in winter and again, using left-overs for lunches is often an effective way of getting more vegetables into every day.

Baking is another very simple way of getting some more vegies into your own and your kids' diets. Extend banana bread and muffin recipes with grated carrot, sweet potato or zuchinni. Chocolate combined with zuchinni or beetroot works very well for healthier cakes and muffins, and pumpkin used in baking, such as pumpkin scones, is also usually very popular, especially as a lunchbox option.

There are lots of good cookbooks out to help with ideas so have a look at some if you need some inspiration to improve your family's intake.

11.3 Go organic if you can

Organic food is often more expensive, but it tastes so much better and is so much better for you. If you can afford it, go the whole way with organic everything including fruit and vegetables, meats, eggs and grains. If that's too expensive, at least try to choose organic fruit and vegies to reduce your exposure to pesticide residues that are present in our supermarket foods at disturbing levels.

The main factor stopping people from choosing organic produce is often financial, as we tend not to prioritise our own health unless we're already sick.

Think hard about the wisdom of saving a dollar now at the expense of your long-term health. It may well be far more economic in the long run to spend a little more on good quality food for your family now and possibly avoid health problems in the future.

Even if you don't put your own health first, think hard about at least sourcing organic produce for your children, especially during the first five years of life. Remember that, dose for weight, children are impacted far more than an adult by the pesticide residues in non organic produce.

Research shows that populations that eat organic food have significantly less (only 10 – 20%) of the residual pesticides in their bodies compared to those who eat regular produce that is pesticide treated. In addition, organic foods have much higher nutrient levels than regular produce, so although you may pay a little more, you get a lot more nutrition from your food.

If you can't stretch to organic fruit and vegetables, at least make sure you wash your produce *really* well to try to limit your intake of contaminants.

11.4 Drink more water

You should aim to drink six to eight glasses of water every day, not including tea and coffee. It should be filtered water if possible.

There is a huge variety of filtration systems available ranging from very inexpensive bench-top jugs to sophisticated reverse-osmosis systems. Find a system that suits your needs, and your budget, and start enjoying the taste and benefits of pure fresh water.

11.5 Eliminate fizzy drinks and cordials

Kids today are drinking an amazing amount of soft drink as part of their normal daily diet. Some kids have a can of Coke or Red Bull every day and several cans on the weekends. While most parents are aware that traditional fizzy drinks such as Coke and Fanta are not supposed to be everyday foods, an incredible number of children also drink cordials, health and sports drinks on a daily basis. What many parents do not realise is that most of these health and sports drinks are just as detrimental to health as regular soft drinks. On the whole they have incredibly high sugar contents – sometimes up to 9 teaspoons per bottle - or even worse they are sweetened by a combination of artificial sweeteners. Most of them also are a cocktail of colours and benzoate preservatives.

Many adults also consume several cans of soft drink a day as part of their normal diet. Aside from the effects of the colours, sweeteners and preservatives contained in them, excessive consumption of cola drinks is also linked to bone deterioration from the leaching of calcium. This is especially worrying in growing children.

These drinks are intended to be consumed occasionally, not every day. Once, they were consumed only at parties or special occasions. Somehow, they have become a feature of our everyday diet. Learn to drink water again, and get your kids drinking water or diluted, additive-free fruit juice.

Water quenches your thirst better than any soft drink will. Keep the soft drink in reserve for parties and special occasions. At the very least, greatly restrict its consumption in your house.

Cordials also are the staple drink of many kids, but they too are full of colours and preservatives of which kids don't need regular daily doses. Again, eliminate them if you can. Replace them with diluted fruit juice or, preferably, water. At the very least, restrict their consumption in your house.

11.6 Choose no-additive juices

Many of us start each day with a glass of fruit juice, but how many of us realise that this healthy start to our day contains several artificial colours and preservatives?

Most of the cheaper fruit-juice-blend drinks containing 35% juice are the worst culprits. Unfortunately, because they are often cheaper, they are the most popular choice for many Mums trying to keep costs down.

Try, instead, to choose 100% juices. These, in the main, don't have colours and preservatives added. If cost is a concern, try diluting them with water to make them go further. Even better, buy a juicer and make your own fresh juices. These taste fantastic and are very good for you.

Small "juice poppers" have become a lunch-box favourite for school kids. Again, most of these contain little fruit juice and lots of colours such as Tartrazine (102), Sunset Yellow (110), Brilliant Blue (133) and preservatives including potassium sorbate (202) and sodium metabisulphite (223). These are all additives linked with undesirable health effects.

You can buy additive-free poppers, or make up a drink of diluted juice or plain water to go in the lunch boxes. The appeal of these poppers is they are a convenient size and kids like them, but don't be a sucker for marketing and trends. Avoid these products, and remove another dose of unnecessary harmful additives from your kids' diet.

11.7 Bread

It is the use of calcium proprionate (282) in bread that is of most concern. As discussed earlier, this additive is linked to a wide range of adverse health effects. It is considered one of the most insidious additives as it's contained widely in one of our staple foods that we all regard as healthy. It affects adults and children but also affects babies exposed through breast milk, resulting in gastric upsets and pain, irritability, constant crying and sleep disturbances.

Unfortunately its use is so widespread that it's getting difficult to find products that don't use it. As of July 2017, both *Brumby's* and *Bakers Delight* advise that their breads don't contain this additive, and some supermarket lines such as *Helga's*, *Noble Rise* and *Burgen* say they also don't use it anymore. On the whole it is relatively easy now to find bread which does not use 282 anymore, but, as discussed previously, its still necessary to double check. Some manufacturers have swapped 282 for sorbate preservatives instead. Both crumpets and muffins seem to commonly contain these other problem preservatives now. Also, some manufacturers have decided to work the labelling law weaknesses and "hide" the calcium propionate by using ingredients such as whey or dextrose. Once again, it's a case of consumer beware and it's easy to be caught out by just glancing at the 282 free label on the front of pack but not bothering to read the actual ingredients panel.

There are, of course, organic varieties readily available in the supermarkets now, which are preservative free but which are often also more expensive. Generally these specialty type breads tend to be less processed and more dense than the light and fluffy supermarket varieties, but are a great option if it fits your budget.

Gluten free breads are also a preferred option for many consumers now. Worldwide there is a confirmed increase in celiac disease, meaning more and more people are discovering they cant tolerate gluten. There is also a corresponding, and as yet unexplained, increase in a condition known as Non Celiac Gluten Sensitivity (NCGS). This food intolerance is serious and effects adults and children. Whilst sufferers do not have true auto immune celiac disease, they do exhibit a range of adverse effect symptoms which are linked to a compromised ability to digest the gluten proteins in grains such as wheat. For this reason the demand for gluten free bread and wheat products is rising rapidly in many countries, including Australia. Unfortunately, many of the substitute ingredients used in gluten free products do not compare taste or texture wise with the real bread products. As a result manufacturers often add in numerous additives to help with improving the taste, texture and shelf life of these usually expensive products. What this means is that gluten free bread usually contains 282 as well as colour additives and a variety of processing aids and vegetable gums to try to make it more like the real thing. If you need to be gluten free, then check your labels very well, or consider baking your own.

So what sort of bread should you buy? It is pretty well accepted that most kids seem to prefer fluffy white bread, but this is the most over-processed bread you can buy, with the least amount of nutrition. Once upon a time, bread was *the staff of life*. Baked from whole grain flour using traditional leavening techniques, old fashioned bread was very dense with nutrition. Today's loaves, however, do not really compare. Where as bread used to take several days to prove, prepare and bake, modern day breads can be baked and packaged ready to go within just a few hours, due to the use of processing aids and enzymes and softening additives.

If you want your bread to be tasty and good for you, breads made with wholegrain flour are a better choice nutritionally, and ideally sourdough loaves are less likely to contribute to food intolerance symptoms. With this in mind, you might like to gradually move your bread choice to a healthier no additive choice, but this doesn't have to mean no more white bread ever! Keep it for a treat and enjoy it when eating out, at celebrations and family gathering, or just limit its consumption in your house from everyday to once a week. Ultimately, its your decision, but, if bread is going to be a feature staple of your diet, then it does make sense to eat more of the healthiest version than the over processed fluffy white stuff that is usually chock full of additives.

A final note about bread is undeclared antioxidants. Old fashioned bread was made of 5 ingredients – flour, yeast, water, salt, sugar – and did not contain vegetable oil as a staple ingredient. Today though many, if not most, supermarket loaves routinely include vegetable oil as an ingredient, and often these oils contain synthetic antioxidants such as 310 – 329. Often these antioxidants are NOT declared on the label, So, if your bread lists vegetable oil on the label, you may need to ring the manufacturer and check, or, find a more authentic bread that has not been baked with vegetable oil as an ingredient.

11.8 Butter, margarine and spreads

Since the 1970s, there's been a sustained awareness campaign to alert consumers to the dangers of excessive fat consumption and links to high cholesterol and heart disease. Since then the consumption of margarines and spreads other than butter have soared, but the rates of heart disease have not come down. Heart disease remains the leading cause of death amongst Australians.

Obviously switching to margarine hasn't been the answer to reduce cholesterol and cardiovascular disease. Why? Because the advice we have been given for the past 50 years has actually been wrong! Most recent scientific opinion has concluded that fat in our diets is not the problem and that fat and cholesterol have been very unfairly vilified for all these years, based upon some very flawed science. Current opinion is leaning towards excessive carbohydrates, especially sugar, being a much bigger problem than the inclusion of healthy fats in our diets in relation to cardiovascular disease. That being the case though, there are still healthy fats and harmful fats and your choice of spreads is an important one to think about in terms of your health.

The truth is that margarine isn't necessarily a healthier food than butter. Margarine is a very unnatural product. It is a *hydrogenated fat.* This is a vegetable oil that has been processed to become saturated and in this process the essential fatty acids are destroyed. What remains is an artificial, solid fat that is very long lasting, great for convenience, but at what cost to our health?

Margarine is high in *trans fatty acids* (TFAs). These are dangerous substances known to contribute to higher cholesterol levels and the formation of carcinogenic substances. Be aware that trans fats aren't just in the margarine you buy, but they are also present in large amounts in just about any processed food containing hydrogenated fat or oil as an ingredient.

Our consumption of these substances has increased 50-fold over the past 20 years, and they are getting very difficult to avoid. If you buy packaged cakes, biscuits, most breads, frozen meals and any commercially fried foods (to name just a few), you'll be consuming large amounts of trans fats in your diet every day.

Unfortunately, even if you do want to read labels to avoid these substances, the labelling in Australia is still not as rigorous as in some other countries in relation to trans fats. In Europe today, trans fats are severely restricted with some countries permitting no more than 0.1% in food products. In some countries, including Denmark and Holland, some of the types of margarine sold in Australia would be outlawed, and anything with trans fatty acids in it must state the levels on the label. In Australia, it's only mandatory for manufacturers to declare the total amount of fat and provide a breakdown of the amount of saturated fat. Manufacturers only have to provide a breakdown of trans fats if there's some claim in respect of cholesterol or trans fats.

In addition to this, margarines also usually contain several preservatives, colours and antioxidants to make them last even longer. The antioxidants used are often the most suspect ones including 310 and 320, and they often don't appear on the label. Some margarines and spreads now even contain flavour enhancers, especially the lite and low salt varieties. As the products have less taste, enhancers are included to improve the flavour.

So in our quest for health over the past 50 years, as a nation we have moved from eating natural fats such as butter, to eating way too much of a totally artificial, very unhealthy substance full of additives and trans fats – namely margarine – because that is what we were told was the right thing to do! Sadly, our health as a nation has paid the price for following what is now being described as one of the biggest nutritional lies in history!

So, in hindsight, it turns out that our ancestors were right all along. What they knew by instinct, science has finally confirmed, and that is that our bodies need good fats to be healthy. What we need to do is choose the right foods, to supply the right sort of fats, in the right amounts to to help our bodies to be healthy.

What we need to do is go back to basics and choose the more natural unadulterated options wherever we can. For those of us who have been so conditioned to fear fat, choosing butter over margarine can be difficult, but butter is definitely a better choice. Some people like the olive oil spreads which do contain modest amounts of healthy monosaturated fats, but the benefits of these good fats are often outstripped by the cocktail of additives which are needed to make these spreads look and taste like butter! If you really don't like butter, maybe just use real olive oil on your sandwich, skip the spread altogether or substitute with avocado, hommus or ricotta cheese as your sandwich spread.

In addition to choosing butter over margarine in moderation, avocados are a great source of health fats to include in your diet, as well as extra virgin olive oil, coconut oil and omega 3 fats found in fish and some plant foods such as chia seeds and flaxseeds. Whilst the official guidelines are still cautious about saturated fat consumption, they are very clear that increasing our consumption of monounsaturated fats and anti-inflammatory omega 3 fatty acids is a good idea for everyone.

Deliberately increasing your consumption of these healthy fats is very easy to do. Ditch the margarine and get some better fats from real foods into your everyday diet. It's not that hard to do, and can only be a good thing for your long term health.

11.9 Low fat and lite products

With soaring obesity rates, it's no surprise that there's a huge consumer interest in products that claim to be low fat or lite. Unfortunately, as with the butter example above, it isn't really a matter of *what* we eat, but rather how *much* we eat of certain foods. People love a quick fix, and nobody really likes dieting or limiting their favourite foods. Really though, the problem isn't with full-fat products such as regular ice cream or biscuits, per se. It is just that, overall, we eat too many high fat, high sugar products, and this is the habit we should be changing.

Low fat and lite products, in general, are very unnatural, highly processed products. Often, to make these products lite, a percentage of the fat content is removed. This means the product doesn't taste as good as its full-fat counterpart, so extra sugar or artificial sweeteners and flavour enhancers are added to make them taste more like the real thing. Reducing fat content often leads to changes in colour or texture also, so artificial colours, thickeners and gums are added to improve the appearance and bulk up a watery low-fat product.

Remember also that a product marketed as low fat or lite doesn't necessarily mean low kilojoule. If they have added more sugar to improve the taste after removing the fat, you may be getting just as many empty kilojoules from the product as you'd have got from eating the same amount of the normal product.

This weight-conscious market is a huge cash cow for food manufacturing companies, as people will believe what a label claims, and not too many read the fine print.

Don't be fooled into believing that low fat or lite necessarily means healthier or better for you.

Eating these highly altered foods often means a much higher intake of unnecessary additives in your diet every day. The smarter thing to do is to try to stick to foods that are as close as possible to their natural state. If you do choose the lite varieties, take the time to find ones that are lite *and* low in additives.

Switching to low fat and lite will not, in itself, cure a weight problem or improve health if the ratio of foods is still out of balance. A healthy diet needs to be high in natural, unprocessed foods and low in sweets and treats. Think about how much of the processed packaged "lite" foods you eat, and concentrate on eating less of them and more fresh fruit, nuts and natural foods.

11.10 Salt

Over the past 30 years, there's also been a great improvement in our awareness about the negative health effects of too much salt in our diets. As a nation we have responded, and studies confirm that we do tend to add less salt to our foods at home than we did 30 years ago, but we are still eating far too much. How can this be? Because we're buying it already added to our foods at the supermarket every week.

Our consumption of processed and packet foods has increased steadily over the past 30 years as a reflection of our busy lives, and we now find that the salt is included in our processed foods in very high concentrations.

The average recommended intake of salt per adult per day is no more than 2.5 grams of sodium. As a guide, one teaspoon of salt has 2 grams of sodium. So, just over a teaspoon of salt per day is the maximum for an adult, and children should have no more than a third of this amount. What we find, though, is that most of us eat far more than that every day and only about a third of what we eat comes from the salt shaker. The rest is hidden in the processed foods that make up a high proportion of our diet.

Sodium contents are surprisingly high in even staple foods such as bread and cheese. Two slices of average wholemeal bread contain about 500 milligrams of sodium, and 30 grams of processed cheddar cheese contains 400 milligrams of sodium, so a child having a cheese sandwich for lunch could be exceeding his daily sodium allowance without eating anything else!
The main culprits, however, are breakfast cereals, canned foods, canned soups, sauces, cooking sauces, flavour bases, packet soups and frozen meals.

It makes a big difference choosing low-salt varieties of products such as baked beans and spaghetti. Half a cup of canned baked beans contains an average of 570 milligrams of salt but a salt reduced variety can contain as little as 40 milligrams. Some pasta stir-through sauces (enough for two servings) contain 2,500 milligrams of salt and most brands of tomato sauce contain 200 milligrams in just one tablespoon.

Breakfast cereals are another area to look at carefully. A recent Health Department survey in Western Australia revealed that a serve of *Rice Bubbles* has a whopping 72 times the sodium level of *Quick Oats*. Frozen foods are another potent source of hidden sodium that varies greatly from brand to brand. *Logan Farm Crinkle Cut Oven Fries* contain only 3 milligrams of sodium per 100 grams; whereas, *Birds Eye Golden Crunch Fries* contain 100 times more.

Unlike the low fat and lite products discussed previously, it makes good sense to shop for no-salt, low salt and salt-reduced products wherever possible, especially for children. Most kids in Australia consume more salt than most adults should have every day. Labels will give you sodium content per 100 grams, so have a look and go for the low-salt choices, preferably those containing no more than 120 milligrams of sodium per 100 grams.

11.11 Sugar

We nibble our way through mountains of sugar every year, and in 2011, Australians consumed on average around 42 kilograms of sugar each, according to the Australian Bureau of Statistics report *Apparent Consumption of Refined Sugar in Australia (1938 – 2011)*.

The World Health Organisation recommends our sugar consumption should only make up five percent of our total calorie intake, which equates to about 25 grams or 6 teaspoons a day. Based on the above statistic of 42 kilograms a year, this means that we are averaging 115 grams per day, or 27 teaspoons of sugar, each, per day.

So although we may have cut down on the amount of sugar we add to our food and drinks, it's sneaking into our diets, pre-mixed for our convenience by the manufacturers. It is in the obvious sources such as biscuits, cakes, yoghurts, ice creams and soft drinks, but also in less obvious sources such as fruit juice, sauces and marinades, mayonnaise, breakfast cereals, canned foods and frozen meals.

The labels will confess to how much sugar is in a product, so if you don't want to eat another 42 kilograms of sugar this year, have a look at what's in your weekly shopping and get rid of the brands with high sugar contents. As an easy guide, remember that 5 grams is about equal to 1 teaspoon of sugar. It doesn't matter at all if it is sucrose, fructose or glucose – it is all still sugar. As a very loose rule, aim for products which contain no more than 15g per 100gm of sugar in total. Some fruit juices and fruit bars are the worst culprits for excess sugar with many popular fruit bars and muesli bars containing up to 15gm of sugar in each 20gm bar!!

Again, just by reverting as much as possible to foods in their most natural state and avoiding processed and packaged products, you'll eliminate many products high in sugar. In the process, you'll be doing your body a huge health favour.

In May 2004, the WA Health Department released a survey of well-known cereals to show how much sugar, salt and fibre are in the most popular brands. The results showed that many popular brands such as *Rice Bubbles* and *Nutrigrain* have incredibly high levels of salt and sugar, despite the public perception created by slick marketing that they are relatively healthy foods.

Have a look at the labels on the packets in your pantry. Inform yourself, and make a better choice next time you go shopping.

11.12   Whole grains

In combination with our over consumption of saturated fats, salt and sugar, as a nation we also don't eat enough whole grains. Our favourite choices are white bread, white rice and pasta. Combined with our under consumption of fresh fruit and vegies, we don't get enough fibre.

The simplest way to introduce more whole grains into your diet is to switch today to wholemeal bread. (Not white bread with grains in it — wholemeal made with wholemeal flour.) It has much more taste that white bread, and kids will get used to it if you insist on the change.

Look also at your breakfast cereals. Many of the most popular brands have almost negligible fibre content and are more confectionary than cereal. This is an easy avenue to increase the dietary fibre intake for the whole family. The best way to do this is to start eating porridge or untoasted muesli for breakfast. (Watch out for high sugar contents in some commercial brands.)

If your family has to stay with the highly processed cereals, at least choose the varieties with the highest fibre and lower salt and sugar contents such as *Weet Bix* and *All Bran*. If you can't get the family to switch completely, at least restrict the rations of the junky brands to once a week or mix some of the higher fibre varieties on top. Just a little bit can make a big difference.

Another good idea is to sprinkle Linseed, Sunflower and Almond mix (LSA) on top of your cereal. This mix is just a combination of ground up nuts and seeds and adds in not only fibre but some much needed healthy fats, vitamins and minerals as well. It is readily available in supermarkets or health food stores or, even better you can easily make your own at home. It is best stored in the fridge to stop the oils from going off. In our house we just gradually introduced a rule that *"sprinkles"* are always added to breakfast cereals to put some nutrition back into them. My kids didn't like them particularly but it did drive home a clear message that the store bought stuff didn't have very much goodness in it. They can also be added easily to smoothies, muffin, cake and cookie mixes for an extra fibre and nutrition boost.

Next, start to eat brown rice instead of white, at least some of the time. It takes a little longer to cook, but it does have a delicious nutty flavour and goes well with all dishes. You can also switch to wholemeal pasta and can start to introduce some legumes into your diet; e.g. chickpeas, beans and lentils. Australians on the whole eat far too few of these highly nutritious, fibre-packed foods, but they are quite easy to incorporate into your diet. Chickpeas and beans (fresh or canned) are great, easy additions to salads, stews and especially curries. Quinoa is another good staple to add into your diet and makes a nice change from rice. It is very easy and quick to cook and packed full of protein and nutrition, and offers almost twice as much fibre as most other grains.

Eat more nuts, dried fruit and seeds (organic if possible). These healthy foods are great for snacks instead of biscuits and snack bars, and provide another easy way to boost your fibre intake. Stay away from breakfast bars and fruit rollups. These are little more than lollies often with up to 60% sugar content.

Finally, just eat more fruit and vegetables every day. The fibre contained in vegetables especially is particularly good for us, and even better when eaten raw. It is so beneficial to get some salads into your weekly meal plan and to make a conscious effort to snack on fruits and vegetables rather than cakes and cookies. I find keeping a container of cut up carrots and celery sticks in the fridge means that we are all much more likely to actually eat them as a snack, usually with some dip such as hommus. Many kids are never offered raw vegetables as a snack option, but often they prefer the crunchy raw vegetables to the cooked ones! A bag of carrot sticks with some grapes,rockmelon or dried fruit is great option for the lunchbox or an after school snack. If you think your kids don't like veggies, maybe just start offering some options regularly (and role model eating them yourself,) and just see what happens. You may get a pleasant surprise as their tastebuds get used to the crunch and taste of real fresh vegies.

Implementing just these simple changes will reap important overall health benefits for your whole family. Even if you don't make a complete change to whole grains, improving by at least 50% on what you do now will be significant.

11.13 Cooking sauces and flavour bases

One of the many by-products of our busier lifestyles has been the advent of the instant cooking sauces and flavour base sachets. The range is huge: *Maggi Cook in the Pot, Chicken Tonight, Dolmio Sauces, Continental Easy Meals, Kantong Stir Through Sauce* and many, many more. Because they make a tasty sauce and because they let us whip up a meal very easily, they are favourites with many people, especially busy families.

Amazingly, though, once these one-pot wonders did not exist, yet families 50 years ago still enjoyed tasty stews, casseroles, pasta, stir fry and curries. How did they do it? Easily, you see, because people used to cook, not just open a packet or jar. If you want to avoid a large source of questionable additives, excessive salt, sugar and harmful oils in your diet, you need to look carefully at your use of these ready-made sauces (and also the instant noodle and pasta sauce products), upon which many of us have come to rely as weekly standards in our diet.

"Oh no", I hear you groan. "That's going to be too hard. I don't have time to make this change! I haven't got time to cook a meal from scratch!" Relax, it's not that hard, and once you have a look at the additives that make some of these products so tasty, I doubt you'll want to be feeding them to your family every night anyway.

Although it's best to cook your own and steer away from these convenience ranges, once again there's good news for those of you who can't imagine cooking dinner without a jar or a packet. Across most of these product ranges, there are again good and bad choices.

Apart from horrific salt levels in a lot of these products, the reason a lot of these products taste so good is because of the heavy use of flavour enhancers 620 to 637. Many also add colours such as Allura red (129), Tartrazine (102) and Annatto (160) all of which have question marks surrounding their long term safety.

You can still keep some of these products in the pantry for emergency standbys and those nights when you just need something quick and easy, but do try to invest a little bit of time to make sure they are the ones with the least amount of harmful additives and ingredients. As a very general rule, most tomato based Italian cooking sauces do not contain harmful additives, but the salt and sugar levels are often much higher than a homemade sauce. Similarly, the taco and Mexican seasoning mixes usually do not contain harmful additives, but the salt levels can be astronomical compared to a homemade seasoning. Many curry type cooking sauces are fine also, although do watch out for tartrazine and other artificial colours which are often snuck into these products to make them look more authentic.

Since this book was first published there has been a big improvement across these products resulting in the removal of MSG and artificial colourings. However, in many cases it has been replaced with legally unlabelled MSG in the form of hydrolysed vegetable protein or similar ingredients which do not demand label disclosure. The take home message here is be aware. Most of the flavour base options or cooking sauces often contain unlabelled MSG and unhealthy levels of salt, sugar, combined with unhealthy fats. Treat these products as convenience foods rather than family staples wherever possible and be aware of what is actually in them. With a little awareness you can still enjoy the convenience of these products, but you can also make sure you avoid exposing your family to numerous servings of suspect additives just by choosing the varieties with the most natural ingredients.

11.14 Two-minute noodles and pasta snacks

Observing people at the checkouts whilst researching this book, I was astounded at the volume of two-minute noodles and similar products many families buy. The bad news is that none of these products are good choices additive wise. Even the noodles themselves are sometimes not okay with many popular brands containing colours and antioxidant 319 in the actual noodles, and the flavour sachets are all laden with MSG, flavour enhancers, colours and salt.

If your kids are hooked on these, start wreaking some changes at your house because these are not good food for anyone, especially not kids.

A tasty and easy alternative is to buy plain noodles made from wheat flour, water and salt. Cook them drain them and gently heat them through with some additive free tomato sauce, sweet chilli sauce or tamari and honey. This might take you three minutes, not two, but it's a much healthier alternative that most kids still enjoy eating immensely. You can also experiment with different types of noodles such as soba noodles, buckwheat noodles and udon noodles all of which are quick to cook and tasty.

Instant pasta sauce meals are also a product range which, on the whole, are chock full of too much salt, flavour enhancers, suspect antioxidants and colours. There are definitely some varieties that are better than others, but these products should be seen as very occasional side dishes, not complete meals, and should not feature as a regular part of your diet. Like two-minute noodles, many people favour these convenient "meals" for the kids under the mistaken impression that they are a relatively healthy choice. They are not.

A far healthier alternative would be to boil some pasta and toss through some cold chicken, tomato, ricotta and grated cheese. This honestly doesn't take any more time than it takes to open the packet and cook it in the microwave, but it's a far superior choice healthwise.

11.15 Avoid processed meats

This is a big one, especially for children who consume probably more processed meats on average in their school lunches every day than most adults. Meats such as ham, polony and salami are all preserved with nitrates or nitrites, which are suspected human carcinogens. Many of them also contain several suspect artificial colours.

Even packaged ham these days sometimes contains flavour enhancers and vegetable gums like Carrageenan 407. Other processed meats like chicken loaf are usually full of flavour enhancers and/or MSG. Aside from the additives in them, the fat and salt contents of these products are very high and they should not be featuring as a substantial part of our everyday diet.

It is easy to make some changes to eliminate or greatly reduce your use of these products. The first thing to do is to limit how many times a week you and your family eat these items. If you have to, give the kids a polony (devon) or ham sandwich once a week, not every day.

Our family used to eat a lot of ham and processed meat but we now buy a small amount every 2 weeks and we enjoy maybe one ham sandwich a fortnight. We also buy low nitrate, organic ham which is available through organic food suppliers and more and more butchers as demand grows.

Instead of processed meat, choose different fillings such as cheese or egg and enjoy the variety. Don't buy the one-kilo knobs of polony as it just sits in the fridge to be snacked on and is gone before you know it.

Next, start to enjoy real the taste and nutrition of cold meat again. An easy habit to start is to use the weekends to cook up a large chicken or a leg of lamb, beef or pork in the oven or slow cooker. Slice it up and keep it in the fridge, ready to use in sandwiches, salads and snacks during the week. Having the meat ready to go means it is also easy to add it to an omelette, stir fry, toasted sandwich or noodle topping for substantial after school snacks. If there is more than you can use keep it sliced up in the freezer. Rotating the choice of meat each week also ensures variety. Real roasted meat sandwiches for lunch are far nicer than polony or artificial chicken roll, and contain far less salt, less fat and no additives. For everyone in the family, this simple change will eliminate a considerable number of unsafe additives from the daily diet.

11.16 Party food

Once you become aware of the number of carcinogens and other questionable substances that are in our food, it's hard to look at a children's party table laden with frankfurts, fairy bread and *Cheezels* the same way. Even as parents who generally try to limit junk intake by their kids, we still allow them to feast on these foods on special occasions such as birthdays, even though we know this food is no good for them. With what you now know, doesn't that seem like a crazy thing to do?

As I researched this book and worked hard to eliminate so many harmful additives from my family's diet, I became determined NOT to do the party additive binge again for my kids and all their friends. My resolve became even firmer after discovering that one of my children suffered asthma attacks after eating certain preservatives and MSG in some "healthy foods" served at a school class party. So, starting from my daughter's third birthday, and for every party since then, we have always enjoyed a delicious spread of additive free party foods, that the children have all enjoyed. These happy parties of well behaved children devouring a table laden with good food have been a pleasure to watch and for me, it has been very convincing that additives in food have a very real and observable effect on many (if not most) children. It makes me happy to send kids home well fed and happy, not hyped up, irritable and wrecked, after all, parties are menat to be fun!

So, the next time you have a kids' party to prepare for, you have a choice. Forget about healthy eating for the day and pump the kids full of hundreds of different additives and anti nutrients, OR, serve up some delicious additive safe foods and treats which the kids will still love, but which you know wont be doing them any harm. Yes, it does take more time to provide home cooked food, but it is usually cheaper in the long run. Even if you decide not to cook from scratch and stay with pre packaged foods, taking the time to find and select the best low additive choices is a really good change to make. Here are some suggestions for some popular tasty alternatives which are easy to do:

- Replace store bought party pies or sausage rolls with homemade sausage rolls using puff pastry and real beef, pork or chicken mince. You can hide some carrot and zuchinni in these very easily. Make them in advance and just re heat on the day when needed. Similarly, mini meatballs are also quick and easy to make in advance and reheat as needed.

- Replace cocktail frankfurts – instead pre cook some additive free sausages (beef, pork or chicken), reheat when needed, sliced up into bite size pieces and served with some dipping sauce and toothpicks for easy, hygienic handling.

- Fairy bread is an old time favourite but the regular sprinkles are a chemical cocktail of artificial colours. Hopper Natural Sprinkle are one example of a safer option available on line, if you want to keep fairy bread on the menu with a clean conscience!

- Old fashioned baking staples such as chocolate crackles, honey joys and pikelets are also always very popular and the kids love making these in preparation for the party. To update chocolate crackles to a healthier version, substitute coconut oil instead of copha and use puffed brown rice instead of rice bubbles.

- Make your own cake if you can. The most basic butter cake or chocolate cake using real flour, eggs and sugar is a huge improvement on a store bought cake full of trans-fats and additives. If you are short of time many bakeries offer a basic sponge which you can take home and decorate.

- For cake decorations go for natural colours instead of the artificial food colours or avoid the colours altogether and go for chocolate or vanilla icing. Instead of decorating the cake with lollies as so many do, perhaps decorate with toys to suit the party theme, such as toy cars, animals, lego figurines or flowers.

- Have lots of healthy real food on the table as well – fruit platters, sandwiches, crackers, cheese, carrot and vegie sticks. You may be surprised how many kids will eat some vegies if they are on offer.

- For drinks for younger children, stick with water and juice – in my experience nothing sends kids into an additive overload more quickly than an overload of soft drink. For a special sparkly drink for older kids mix juice with lemonade to add some colour and bubbles.

- For lolly bags, just don't go overboard, especially for the younger kids. If it is your tradition to send home lolly bags, select some additive safe favourites such as Freddo Frogs, Maltezers or Natural Confectionary Company snakes, jellies and jubes. Instead of lots of lollies maybe provide some novelties such as bouncy balls, bubbles or balloons along with a thankyou note.

Simple changes such as these will go unnoticed by your children. They will still have a great time and enjoy their party, and you may well find you have a great sense of satisfaction and some very grateful parents at the end of your next party

11.17   Foods for young children

As parents, one of the most important things we can do for our children is to set them up with healthy eating habits from an early age. This means starting from the time of their first foods and continuing the good choices throughout their childhood.

Most women are extremely careful about what they eat and drink during pregnancy and breastfeeding to protect their baby. Unfortunately, however, as children grow and start to eat a wider variety of foods, parents often unwittingly make some very poor choices. Many of these choices are guided by the aggressive marketing of the food manufacturers that convince us that their products are good healthy choices for our children when, in fact, they are not. Their marketing makes us feel good about their foods when, in fact, their food may be damaging our children's health.

We have discussed earlier the negative effects of substances like MSG and Aspartame, and the ability of these additives to impact the developing foetus. These additives are capable of causing damage to the brain development of young animals and disrupting the endocrine (hormone) system later in life. As such, they should be *avoided by women during pregnancy and breastfeeding, and should not be fed to young children at all.*

The human brain continues to grow for three years after birth, and there are many critical phases of development throughout this time.

Unfortunately, from the age of two, or even younger in some cases, children are being allowed to eat foods containing these substances regularly. Foods such as chips, savoury biscuits, flavoured rice crackers, tinned meals, processed meats, instant noodles and pasta snacks feature prominently in many children's diets. These same foods are promoted as good choices by food manufacturers.

Even worse, these products are often made more appealing to parents through the use of convenient kid-size packaging. *You cannot rely on the food manufacturers to tell you what's good for your child.* Take a stand. Take charge of your children's health, and stop buying these products for your kids. They are definitely not good for them nutritionally, and they may well be doing them real, long-term harm.

Remember when starting your child on solid food, that you have a blank canvas to work with. It is very much within your control to shape your child's tastes and eating habits for the rest of their life. Don't add salt or sugar to any of their foods as their tastebuds are very sensitive. Even if their food appears bland to you, it will taste great to them just as it is.

Cook your own baby food using organic ingredients if possible, and only use tinned baby foods for occasional meals if you have to. There are organic varieties of baby food readily available in supermarkets and health-food stores, so choose them if you can to avoid your baby eating products containing pesticide residues.

Be very careful also of any baby foods with *vegetable oils* listed as an ingredient as some may contain antioxidants which aren't on the label. During the research for this book I discovered that a leading brand of baby food had previously contained antioxidant 320 in many of its products that contained vegetable oil. This additive is *specifically banned in foods for infants and young children* in Australia, because it is a known carcinogen and xenoestrogen, yet it had been in circulation in these baby-food products for many years!

This manufacturer now advises that, their products no longer contain any vegetable oil and therefore no antioxidant 320. This is good, but the question remains: *why this was allowed to go on for so long?*

As your baby grows and you start to introduce more foods, stay well clear of the high additive, high trans fats, processed foods that many kids get hooked on from the age of about two.
In particular, be wary of junky breakfast cereals, MSG-laden savoury biscuits, chips, rice crackers, two-minute noodles, pasta snacks with MSG, popper fruit-juice drinks, brightly coloured

foods, white bread and processed meats. These are not good foods for anyone, but especially not for young children.

Even if your child is already eating these things, you can gradually improve their diet. You are the parent; you are in charge. Just make changes slowly, one at a time, and you'll gain a great sense of satisfaction as you make the healthy changes and watch your child start to enjoy real food once again.

11.18   Smarter rewards

If you are a parent, it can be very helpful to take a moment and think about how you tend to motivate your kids in relation to food. Do you condition them to see a trip to McDonalds or a candy bar as a treat? Don't worry, you are not alone! Most parents I know resort to food bribery as a default position which often gets great results! However, if you do reward and motivate your kids with unhealthy food, just be aware that this dynamic often becomes a regular habit which sends very mixed messages to your children about the consumption of unhealthy foods

Instead, you can choose to consciously educate your kids that these types of "food" choices are treats which taste good, but really do our bodies no good and really need to be kept for occasional treats. Talk about the benefits of fresh, live foods which nourish our bodies as compared to the consequences of eating processed, fake foods which, although they may taste good, have no real goodness in them and which make our bodies feel sluggish and unhealthy.

That's not to say you have to swear off take away and treats – not at all! But take the opportunities as they arise to help your kids understand the place of fast food and treats in the diet, and be realistic about how much is too much. A lot of Australian families are in denial about how much fast food they eat. According to a CSIRO Report published in 2014, Australians were eating three times more junk food than the recommended daily intake, with many families consuming fast food every day, rather than as an occasional indulgence

Many of us have grown up with the same poor conditioning, and we pass it on to our kids without even thinking about it.

However, if you have young children, you can change the pattern. If you wish to reward or motivate your child, think of rewards other than fast food or lollies. Maybe they can choose an exotic piece of fruit from the greengrocers, a fresh soft bun from the bakery, or a muffin from the health food store.

Even better, get food out of the equation and reward them with a small toy or a book or, better still, *your time*. For young children, this is what they want most anyway.

Reward them with an extra story, a trip to the park or 15 minutes of your undivided attention to play whatever game they choose. Even if your kids already see fast food and junk food as treats, you can start to "recondition" them just by using these rewards less often and introducing new healthier rewards for your family to enjoy.

You can still buy lollies and treats and take away for kids if you want to – of course you can! However, you have the capacity now to apply your knowledge of safer additives to guide your product selections. For example, choose a plain white or chocolate Freddo Frog rather than one with the coloured fillings, and avoid several coal tar dyes with your chocolate. If you like McDonalds milkshakes, choose vanilla or chocolate over strawberry so you don't choose a sneaky serving of Allura Red, Brilliant Blue and Tartrazine. Simple changes such as these are easy to implement and will help to prevent a lot of unnecessary, undesirable additives sneaking into your family's diet. When you are out trying to have fun, you don't want the event to be ruined by an additive induced, argument, hyperactivity or meltdown, yet sadly this happens to so many families, so often. Usually the sugar gets blamed, but it is much more likely to be the multiple doses of colours, preservatives and flavour enhancers in the food that you have just paid good money for. Be selective. Treat your family with good quality foods and treats and enjoy the experience of eating out in harmony again!

11.19   Reset your bliss point

Within the food manufacturing industry, there's a term known as the *bliss point*. This refers to enhancing the taste intensity of product to a point that just makes you want to eat more and more. Immediate examples that spring to mind are some corn chips, potato chips and savoury biscuits. Once you start eating them, it's hard to stop.

For all of us, our bliss points are being cranked up higher and higher the more MSG and flavour enhancers we consume. As we eat more artificially flavoured, super-tasty food, we get to like the taste and we go back for more. After a while, normal food tastes bland, so our preferences steer away from natural food to flavour enhanced foods.

Our children's bliss points are being determined at a very early age by the foods they eat, and they are growing up unable to enjoy the taste of plain, healthy food because they have been weaned onto highly flavoured foods from a very early age.

Once you eliminate or greatly reduce your consumption of MSG and other flavour enhancers, you'll be surprised how quickly your bliss point resets itself. High MSG foods that you once used to enjoy and devour in excess will no longer have the same appeal, and you'll find that their taste is too salty and over the top. It really does happen quite quickly once you cut out these additives from your diet. Try it and see for yourself.

The same applies to kids too. If you cut out these foods from their diet, they will complain at first, but stick with it and you'll be amazed that in a very short time they are perfectly happy with plain potato chips or lightly salted corn chips, or additive free rice crackers, rather than MSG laden chips and additive heavy savoury biscuits. This might be hard to imagine, but it will happen once you regain control of your own bliss point and reprogram your kids' tastebuds back to a level closer to that which nature intended.

Chapter 12: Get to it: take control of your kitchen

12.1 Introduction

If you live alone then it's simple to make whatever changes you like to your diet and eating style whenever you like. You only have yourself to consider. If, however, you're a parent or spouse who has to make decisions about what everyone in the family eats, balancing those decisions with everyone's likes and dislikes, it becomes a little more complicated to implement change and maintain a happy household.

Remember, though, ultimately it's *your* kitchen, and if you're the one expected to shop and cook for everyone then you have a big say about these decisions. If you have no kids but your spouse isn't supportive of the changes you want to make, that's fine. Just go ahead and implement the changes you feel are important, and let them shop and cook for themselves for a while. I guarantee you that it won't last long and they will either end up happily eating the healthier low-additive meals you provide, or you'll have half as much shopping and cooking work to do!

If you have children to shop and cook for, though, you may have to prepare yourself for a bit of a battle at first to implement the changes. Even from a very young age, children develop very strong likes and dislikes and are capable of waging sustained defiance campaigns against changes they don't like. Just remember: your children's health and wellbeing is your responsibility. You are the adult and, for quite some time to come, you do know best.

Remember too, that it's one of the most important functions of parenting to lay down good eating habits that will steer your children towards long-term good health. We really only have total control of this area for a few short years. Once they start school, they are influenced from many other directions, and if you cannot gain good control over their eating habits before then, it's going to be extremely hard to instil positive changes down the track.

Many parents have found this when confronted with a health problem such as excess weight, asthma or allergies requiring diet change in the older child. It can be very difficult to undo bad habits that have been laid down in early childhood. If you can instil good patterns before they go to school, you'll be doing their long-term health a huge favour. *We need to prioritise our children's health now, not wait for the problems to emerge later on.*

Take the time though to explain your decisions regarding food, even to very young children. From a very young age toddlers can understand and accept the concepts of healthy and unhealthy foods, and the need to eat well to be strong and healthy. You aren't negotiating, just explaining why the changes are being made. In the process, you are teaching them the foundations for healthy eating patterns and giving them a chance to develop an understanding and a taste for real food which will be with them throughout their life.

For little children, it's probably easier as they have no other source of income or food. Implement your changes *gradually,* and stick as close as possible to their favourites. Just substitute low-additive varieties and gradually introduce new foods and habits such as more fruit and vegetables, whole grains and healthier cereals.

By going low additive there are certainly individual products that you'll no longer buy, but you can still eat the same sort of food, just better choices. The kids may fuss and carry on for a short time, but dig your heels in and be firm, and it will soon pass. Your family's tastes will very quickly adjust too. Before you know it, the changes will be made and any fuss and bother about it will be a distant memory.

For older children, it's a little more difficult as you cannot control what they spend their pocket money on and what they eat at school. The best advice here is to lead by example and explain to them what you're doing and why. Give them this book to read and take them shopping with you to help pick the best low-additive choices while still enjoying the sorts of food they are used to.

Involve them in cooking and experimenting with recipes without additives which still taste great and, in the process, develop some new favourite family meals. If it makes life easier, you might want to agree to just dramatically reduce some items rather than eliminate them totally from your pantry. For example, you may agree to buy only one bottle of soft drink a week, and decide that it's only drunk on weekends. Agree that one night a week they can cook whatever they like for tea. Don't criticise or try to influence what they choose, even if you don't want to eat it yourself.

Involving older children in setting the framework for the new eating plan is much more likely to succeed than trying to impose unilateral changes "for their own good".

You have to accept that, even if you eliminate the worst additives from your home, your teenager will still probably snack on MSG-laden chips and Coke on the way home from school (possibly for no other reason than just to defy you!), and there's nothing you can do about that. Just be happy in the knowledge that when at home they eat healthy food and they are now eating much less of these harmful additives overall. The 80/20 rule (or the 90/10 rule if you prefer), is a good guide to go by. Unless you have serious food allergies and intolerances you don't need to be fanatical about food. However, if you strive to follow your additive safe food plan 80 – 90 per cent of the time, you are doing a great job and you will get there. Whilst it can seem overwhelming at first, adopting this philosophy can really help you to relax and approach your changes gradually and successfully.

Before you start, you may want to take a moment and write down a sample menu for a week of what you and your family eat now for all meals and snacks. Put it away in a safe place then, in six months, after you have made your changes, review it against what your family is eating then.

You may be amazed at the changes, extremely happy at the amount of additives you have eliminated, and astounded at some of the food you used to eat and enjoy, which you now never crave and can't imagine ever buying again.

If you reflect on the general health of your family at the same time, you may well be surprised to find a significant improvement in everybody's health, behaviour and mood.

Have a look now at the following additive-consumption comparison tables to see just how easy it is to make a huge difference to your overall additive intake, just by applying all that you have learnt, shopping smarter and choosing the lower-additive products available in the supermarket.

12.2   Additive consumption comparison

The following tables have been prepared to illustrate clearly how easily the average person can consume large doses of additives as part of an everyday diet. Just by shopping smarter, you can select the lower additive products available in the shops and quite dramatically reduce you consumption of all additives, especially those with known or suspected adverse health effects.

The tables compare two similar variations on the menu below, but menu 2, The Additive Alert Menu, highlights just how easy it is to avoid additive laden products without changing your food selections greatly. For the purpose of this example I have only included like for like prepacked foods, and, for this reason, some of the "safer" choices do still contain some additives. The additive count for the Additive Alert menu could easily be reduced to zero, simply by replacing some items with home made alternatives. This menu is in no way offered as a " good" example of healthy eating. It is purely intended to illustrate how quickly additives add up in our everyday diets, and how simple product selection choices can either boost or reduce your daily intake of additives. The additives attributed to each product were taken direct from the product labels and were correct at the time the research was undertaken. However, companies can and do change their formulations from time to time in response to consumer demands, so, always remember – consumer beware – and check your labels from time to time to see if anything has changed!

Additives listed in bold in the following tables have known or suspected adverse health implications. For specific details refer to the Additive Effects table provided at Appendix 4.

Ok – so what's on the menu?

Breakfast
Cereal
Toast with spread and jam
Orange juice

Morning Tea
Yoghurt tub
Biscuits

Lunch
Chicken ,cheese and salad wrap
Strawberry milk drink

Dinner
Chicken cooked with simmer sauce
Apple pie and vanilla icecream

Now, lets break that down and compare and see exactly where the additives are hiding.

Breakfast: Standard menu

Breakfast	Total Additives on label	Number of Suspect Additives
Uncle Toby's Honey Cheerios	**508** 511 **150** 160b	3
Buttercup Country Split Bread	481 471 **472e 282**	2
Country Gold Soft and Light Butter	440 322 470 471 **202 160b 320**	3
Cottees Raspberry Conserve Diet	1200 440a 401 **407** 330 331 **951** 202	3
Daily Juice Co Orange Drink	330 300 **202 211 160b**	3
Totals	**28 Additives**	**15**

Breakfast : Additive Alert Menu

Breakfast	Total Additives on label	Number of Suspect Additives
Uncle Toby's Oat Flakes	0	0
Mainland Butter Soft	0	0
St Dalfour Raspberry Jam	0	0
Crusta Orange Juice Preservative Free	0	0
Totals	**0 Additives**	**0**

Morning Tea: Standard Menu

Morning Tea	Total Additives on label	Number of Suspect Additives
Nestle Diet Yoghurt Juice Nectarine	441 **950** 415 412 440 **951 296 202 160b 120** 509	6
Arnotts Tim Tam Chewy Caramel	322 476 422 471 322 **102 110 129 133 150** 503 500	5
Totals	**23 Additives**	**11**

Morning Tea: Additive Alert Menu

Morning Tea	Total Additives on label	Number of Suspect Additives
Margaret River Dairy Co Mango and Passionfruit Yoghurt	0	0
Arnotts Monte Chocolate Biscuit	322 476 500	0
Totals	**3 Additives**	**0**

Lunch: Standard Menu

Lunch	Total Additives on label	Number of Suspect Additives
Mission Spinach and Herb Wrap	**320 450** 500 **102 133** 471 412 **466** 297 **282 200**	7
Kraft Sweet Chilli Mayonnaise	**1403** 1412 1422 415 330 **320** 124 **101** 160a	4
Country Gold Soft and Light Butter	440 322 470 471 **202 160b 320**	3
Don Chicken Breast Meat	326 262 **407 451** 450 **508 452**	4
Kraft Free Singles Cheese Slice	339 341 **220 160b 171 200**	4
Masters Strawberry Milk	**122 124 102**	3
Totals	**43 Additives**	**25**

Lunch: Additive Alert Menu

Lunch	Total Additives on label	Number of Suspect Additives
Kal's Flat Bread Wrap	0	0
SW Whole Egg Mayonnaise	0	0
Mainland Butter Soft	0	0
Makers Choice Lightly Smoked Chicken	**223**	1
Mainland Light and Tasty Cheese Slice	0	0
Brownes Dairy Strawberry Milk	0	0
Totals	**1 Additive**	**1**

Dinner: Standard Menu

Dinner	Total Additives on label	Number of Suspect Additives
Leggos Italian Chicken Scallopini Simmer Sauce	410 1441 415 **251 621 627 631** 270 471 **433**	5
Peters No Added Sugar Vanilla Icecream	1200 **420 477** 471 412 341 **160b 955 950**	5
Homebrand Family Apple Pie	**202 223** 471 322 307 1442 450 500 330 **160b**	3
Totals	**29 Additives**	**13**

Dinner: Additive Alert Menu

Dinner	Total Additives on label	Number of Suspect Additives
Masterfoods Creamy Chicken and Mushroom Simmer Sauce	1442 270	0
Peters Original vanilla Icecream	477 471 412	0
Nannas Apple Crumble	1422 500 297 330 410	0
Totals	**10 Additives**	**0**

Let's compare the total number of additives in the two menus:

Standard Menu	Additive Alert Menu
Total Additives = 123	Total Additives = 14
Total number of suspect additives = 64	Total number of suspect additives = 1

We have reduced the total number of additives in the menu from 123 to 14: a reduction of 89% less additives overall!

Better still, we have reduced the total of additives which are linked to adverse health effects from 64 down to just 1 - a reduction of 98%!

(The only reason there was one suspect additive included in the Additive Alert menu is because I couldn't find a single brand of processed chicken meat which did not contain a preservative, as by law cold meat does have to contain preservative). However, simply replacing that item at lunch with some cold home cooked meat from the night before would mean that the entire days menu would not have contained a single suspect additive.

So, you can see quite clearly from this simple example just how easy it is to consume a large number of additives in an average day. With 123 additives in this day alone, it is easy to visualise where our estimated 5 kilograms of additives comes from over a year.

Conversely, I hope this example also shows you just how easy it is to dramatically reduce your consumption of additives, especially those with adverse health links, with very little effort, just by shopping smarter and choosing the lower additive alternatives, or, even better, by rethinking the packaged convenience products and gradually replacing them with more natural and homemade alternatives.

Chapter 13: Taking it further by forcing change

If we as consumers want to have our voices heard, there are two main avenues of action open to us. The first is to vote loudly and decisively with our shopping dollars by supporting strongly those manufacturers who supply products with no harmful additives. While we're doing this, the other companies will see their market share dwindle and will start to question why. It won't take them long to work it out. This is probably the most effective method of forcing change as it centres around impacting company profit — and companies watch over and guard their bottom line ferociously.

Voting with your shopping dollar is far more effective, though, when used in conjunction with letter writing or phone calls to tell companies why we're not supporting their products. If you're making a call to check on antioxidants or other hidden additives in a product and you find that a product contains an unsafe additive, tell the operator that you'll not be buying their product because of the additives they use. This information goes back up the line, especially if this type of feedback becomes more and more common, rather than just an occasional call from some poor person with food allergies.

Manufacturers need to be made aware that it's not just people with actual illnesses or allergies who don't want to eat these chemicals. Everyday, normal, healthy people who are interested in their long-term health and wellbeing also don't want to eat these chemicals, and we need to get this message across. Demand the use of safer alternatives. If enough of us do it, we may see more and more use of the good additives and less and less of the cheap and nasty alternatives that many companies use at the moment.

Sadly, Australia is lagging well behind the trends of many other countries, especially the UK and Europe. Ask anyone who has visited these countries recently and they will confirm that the availability and abundance of additive safe and organic produce is truly startling in comparison to Australia, where such products are often difficult to source and prohibitively expensive to buy. Consumer awareness in Europe about the problems associated with some food additives has driven the manufacturers to take the lead, regardless of what the law demands of them. Following the release of the Southhampton study in September 2007, large manufacturers including Sainsbury's, Tescos and Marks and Spencers were proactive in voluntarily removing many suspect additives from their products, and consumers in the UK consequently have a much easier time finding mainstream groceries that are free from harmful additives.

This should be happening here also, so why is it not? Simply, because manufacturers here are yet to be convinced that this issue is of big enough concern for consumers. It is all about bottom dollar for them and if we consumers are happy to continue to buy products that contain cheap and possibly nasty ingredients, then why would the manufacturers go to the trouble of using more expensive, safer options? Seeing as our regulator is NOT regulating on our behalf, it is unfortunately up to us to drive this change, and we need to do this by communicating directly with the major manufacturers at the checkout, via their feedback lines and though our coordinated lobbying efforts.

The second avenue towards forcing change is to apply sustained pressure on the regulatory authority — in this case Food Standards Australia New Zealand — to change the legislation and protect consumers, as it should. Although it would be nice to imagine that with consumer pressure we could influence FSANZ to ban the use of any food additive with known or suspected adverse health impacts in our food, this isn't a realistic aim in the short term.

However it is totally realistic to believe that with enough consumer pressure we can achieve one very important and fundamental change: *full disclosure in labelling.*

It would be a huge victory for consumers to get rid of the 5% loophole in our legislation, which currently works to the manufacturers' advantage and leaves us in the dark as to what's really in our food. This would be and is the most achievable reform to aim for in the short term.

So how do we make this happen? Simply writing to FSANZ and telling them what we want will be a great start. If FSANZ receives several thousand letters all asking for the same basic change, they will be hard pressed to come up with a compelling reason why it can't be done, especially given that their mandate is *"to protect the health and safety of the people".*

If this is something you'd like to see happen, we've made it easy for you to be part of the process of forcing positive change. At the back of the book is a letter you can use to have your voice heard and demand that FSANZ change the labelling laws to ensure that manufacturers must identify *all* additives in *all* ingredients, no matter how small the percentage.

Either fill in your name and address and sign the letter "as is", or feel free to write your own if you want to say more. For the campaign to be effective, it's critical, though, that all letters consistently ask for the same basic change; i.e. *full disclosure of additives in all ingredients.*

Although it would be nice to demand numerous improvements and changes, to have the maximum chance of success we need to concentrate on one small step at a time.

It would be a powerful start if consumer power could, at the very least, force manufacturers to tell us honestly what's in the food we eat and, thereby, give us the freedom to truly choose what we do and don't wish to eat. This would be a great first step. *If you want to see this happen too, make sure you send off your letter and get your family and friends to do the same by photocopying it or logging onto the website where an electronic version of the petition is available.*

The more letters FSANZ receive asking for the same thing, the harder it will be for them to not act.

Go to it. Let's make a change that counts!

Be aware also that this campaign for truth in labelling is much, much bigger than just the readers of this book. There is a very active campaign for full disclosure in labelling both here in Australia and internationally, and many other countries are far more progressive than Australia.

By sending in this letter, you're not only having your opinion heard, but you'll be supporting a well established push for our rights as consumers to be protected by the agency whose mandate it is to do so.

For more details on other sources associated with truth in labelling, see *Appendix 3, Useful Contacts.*

Appendix 1: Additives to avoid

Suspected carcinogens

These additives have proven or strongly suspected links to cancer in animals and/or humans.

110 122 123 124 127 129 131 132 133 153 155

249 250 251 252

310 319 320 321

407 407a 431 432 433 435 436 466

553

900 914 943a 950 951 952 954 1201

Additives not recommended for children

Pregnant and breastfeeding women may wish to avoid these also.

102 104 110 120 122 123 124 127 129 131 132 133 142 151 153 155
160b 162
211 216 220 221 222 223 224 225 228 249 250 251 252 264 280 281
282 283 290 296
310 311 312 319 320 321 349 355
405 407 407a 420 421 431 432 433 435 436 466
508 514 553 554 555 556
620 621 622 623 624 625 627 631 635 641
914 943a 943b 944 950 951 952 954 955 956 957 966 967
1201 1520 1521

Prohibited in foods for infants and young children by FSANZ guidelines

Children, pregnant and breastfeeding women may wish to avoid these.

249 250 251 252
310 311 312 320 321
420 421
621 627 631 635

Hyperactive or hypersensitive reaction possible

These should be avoided by children, especially those with ADD or ADHD, or anyone with known chemical sensitivities.

102 103 104 110 120 122 123 124 127 129 131 132 133 142 150 151
155 160b
210 211 220 282
319 320 321
421
620 621 627 631 635
951

Previoulsy banned in other countries

These additives are still permitted in Australia despite having been previously banned in other countries, often because of their links to cancer, birth defects or other serious adverse effects demonstrated in animal studies.

102 104 110 120 122 123 124 127 129 132 133 142 151 153 155 173
174 175
320 385
635
952 954

Linked to asthma

These additives have been known to trigger or exacerbate asthma attacks in sufferers. Asthmatics or anyone at risk of asthma may wish to avoid them.

102 104 110 120 122 123 124 127 129 131 132 133 142 151 155
160b 163
200 201 202 203 210 211 212 213 216 220 221 222 223 224 225 228
249 250 251 252 280 281 282 283
310 311 312 319 320 321
407 407a
620 621 622 623 624 625 627 631 635
928 951
1403 1404

Safety suspect: adverse reaction possible

These additives vary greatly in the severity of the associated health concerns. In some cases, the jury is still out about their long-term safety. Other additives in this category are linked to severe effects in existing references. Refer to Additive Effects on page 140 for more info on each additive and the associated health concerns.

100 102 104 110 120 122 123 124 127 129 131 132 133 142 150 151
155 160b 172 173 174 175
200 201 202 203 210 211 212 213 216 218 220 221 222 223 224 225
228 235 249 250 251 252 264 280 281 282 283 290 296
310 311 312 319 320 321 337 338 349 355 385
405 407 407a 409 413 414 416 420 421 422 431 445 466 477 480
482 491
508 510 512 514 519 530 541 553 554 555 556 579
620 621 622 623 624 625 627 631 635 641
914 924 928 943a 943b 944 951 952 954 955 956 965 966 967
1201 1422 1520 1521

<table>
<tr><td>Not recommended for those with salicylate intolerance</td></tr>
<tr><td>

102 104 110 120 122 123 124 127 132 133 142 150 151 155
211 212 213 216 218
310 311 312 321
621 623 627

</td></tr>
</table>

<table>
<tr><td>Not recommended for those with kidney or liver problems</td></tr>
<tr><td>

172 181
201 202 203 211 220 228 252 261
310 336 337 380 385
420 421 450 450a 451 452
508 510 511 514 518 519 554 555 556
622
914 951 952 954 955 956 1201 1520

</td></tr>
</table>

<table>
<tr><td>Recently added to Australian standards
Little information about safety is available for these additives.</td></tr>
<tr><td>

127 143 150 160d 160e 164 173 174 175
242
354 359 363 368
407a 431 445 472f
530 555 560 580 586
635 640 641
914 943a 943b 944 946 953 955 956 957 960 961 962 965 966 967 968 999(i) 999(ii)
1001 1451 1521 1522

</td></tr>
</table>

Appendix 2: Consumer information lines

COMPANY	PHONE
Arnott's	1800242492
Birds Eye	1800061270
CC's Corn Chips	1800501441
Campbells	1800663366
Cerebos Foods	1800656115
Coles	1800061562
Continental	1800888997
Copperpot Dips	(08)82817710
Cottees	1800244054
Crisco Oils	1800638112
Devondale	1800032479
Dolmio	1800816016
Dorata	1800688771
Doritos	1800025789
Farmland	1800061562
Flora	1800628400
Four and Twenty	1800061279
Gold n Canola	1800638112
Greens	1800803605
Heinz Watties	1800037058
Herbert Adams	1800061279
I&J	1800061279
John West	1800888119
Kellogg's	1800000474
Kettle Chips	1800806128
Kraft	1800033275
Lean Cuisines	1800025361
Lowan	1800355718
McCain	1800065521

COMPANY	PHONE
Maggi	1800025361
Masterfoods	1800816016
Mainland	1800032479
Meadow Lea	1800638112
Mills and Wares	(08)93373222
Miracle	1800677807
Nannas	1800061279
Nestle	1800025361
Olive Grove	1800638112
Olivio Bertolli	1800628400
Pampas	1800628883
Pauls	1800676961
Tandaco	1800656115
Safcol	1800819785
Sanitarium	1800673392
Sara Lee	1800650056
Sea Lord	1800061279
Signature Range	1800880078
Smiths	1800025789
SPC	1800805168
Streets	1800643336
Taings	1800682464
Westons	1800643287
White Wings	1800025768
Woolworths WA	(08)93515222

Appendix 3: Useful contacts

Additive Alert: Your Guide to Safer Shopping

We welcome comments and feedback for future editions from consumers and manufacturers alike. Please feel free to e-mail us at additivealert@bigpond.com

Food Standards Australia New Zealand
www.foodstandards.gov.au

This is the regulatory body in Australia and New Zealand that controls the use of food additives in our food as per the *Food Standards Code*.

PO Box 7186
Canberra ACT 2610

Phone: (02) 6271 2222
Fax: (02) 6271 2278

E-mail: Information Officer: info@foodstandards.gov.au

Food Intolerance Network
www.fedup.com.au

This is a NSW-based organisation providing support and assistance for people with food-intolerance issues. This is an excellent and well-maintained information site with a wealth of detail about the effects of food additives on both adults and children. It also provides scientific references in relation to the effects of many food additives. You can subscribe to the free *Failsafe* newsletter, which highlights current issues, research, product updates, recipes and support forums around the country.

E-mail: sdengate@ozemail.com.au

Campaign for Truth in Medicine

www.campaignfortruth.com

This is a UK-based organisation committed to the distribution of accurate health and treatment information from properly researched sources that lead citizens to informed choices. Free monthly newsletter is available about toxins and chemicals in food, personal care and household products. They also have a good online selection of books about a variety of associated topics, especially avoiding toxins and chemicals in daily life.

Campaign for Truth In Labelling

www.truthinlabeling.org

This is a US-based organisation dedicated to the full disclosure of the presence of MSG in all its forms in all foods and personal-care products. They have lots of interesting information and research articles about the effects of MSG and it's unlabelled cohorts such as hydrolysed vegetable protein.

Diabetes Australia

www.diabetesaustralia.com.au

This is a not-for-profit organisation dedicated to minimising the impact of diabetes on Australian society. They are involved in education and awareness strategies and the development of national policies to combat the rising incidence of the disease. This is an excellent resource site for those with diabetes or anyone interested in learning more about the disease, its management and prevention.

Centre for Science in the Public Interest

www.cspinet.org

This US-based nutrition advocacy group has an interesting website that covers a wide range of issues relating to food safety, regulation and labelling in the US. They also publish an award winning newsletter called *Nutrition Action Health Letter* that you can subscribe to and view back copies of online.

Sucralose Toxicity Information Centre
www.holisticmed.com/splenda/

This site presents facts about the artificial sweetener Splenda.

Aspartame (Nutrasweet) Toxicity Information Centre
www.holisticmed.com/aspartame/

This site provides detailed scientific and general documents relating to the toxicity of Nutrasweet, Equal, Diet Coke and other Aspartame containing items.

Asthma Foundations
www.asthmaaustralia.org.au

Freecall 1800 645 130 to enquire about support services and resources in your area.

Australian Breastfeeding Association
www.breastfeeding.asn.au

The Australian Breastfeeding Association is an organisation of people interested in the promotion and maintenance of breastfeeding.

Dr Joseph Mercola
www.mercola.com

Homepage for US-based Dr Joseph Mercola, author of the Total Health Program. Subscribe for his weekly newsletter which contains up-to-date comment on health issues and a great reference site for all health-related questions.

The Parents' Jury

www.parentsjury.com.au

The parents' jury is a web-based network of parents who wish to improve the food and physical activity environments for children in Australia. The Parents' Jury is a forum for parents to voice their views on children's food and physical activity issues, and to collectively advocate for the improvement of children's food and physical activity environments (for example, reduced marketing targeted at young children, more healthy choices for school canteens, and making neighbourhoods safer and more child friendly). Subscribe for their regular newsletter to keep up to date with issues relating to childhood obesity and diabetes.

Appendix 4: Additive effects

#	NAME	ADVERSE REACTION
100–199		
100	Curcumin or Turmeric	Derived from the Turmeric plant root but not the same thing as the common spice Turmeric – can also be produced artificially. Generally regarded as safe for use in foods, but some sources list concerns over long-term safety. Regard with caution – occasional use recommended as safe.
101	Riboflavin or riboflavin 5'-phosphate sodium	
102	Tartrazine	Linked to hyperactivity, skin rashes, migraines, behavioural problems, thyroid problems, and chromosome damage. Previously banned in Norway and Austria.
103	Alkanet or Alkannin	Linked to hyperactivity.
104	Quinoline yellow	Linked to hyperactivity, skin rashes, asthmatics should avoid. Previously banned in USA and Norway - previously banned in Australia.
110	Sunset yellow FCF	Suspected carcinogen, allergies, hyperactivity, upset stomach, skin rashes, kidney tumours, and chromosomal damage. Previously banned in Norway.
120	Carmines or Carminic acid or Cochineal	Red dye derived from a beetle. Commonly linked to hyperactivity, some studies suggest possibly toxic to embryo.
122	Azorubine or Carmoisine	Suspected carcinogen, mutagen, skin rashes, oedema, and hyperactivity. Previously banned in Sweden, USA, Austria and Norway.
123	Amaranth	Suspected carcinogen, mutagen, linked to hyperactivity, asthma and eczema. Previously banned in USA (1976), Russia, Austria, Norway and others.
124	Ponceau 4R	Suspected carcinogen, linked to hyperactivity and asthma. Previously banned in USA and Norway.

#	NAME	ADVERSE REACTION
127	Erythrosine	Suspected carcinogen, linked to thyroid abnormality, brain dysfunction, hyperactivity, and light sensitivity. Previously banned in Norway.
129	Allura Red AC	Suspected carcinogen, skin rashes, hypersensitivity. Previously banned in Denmark, Belgium, France, Germany, Switzerland, Austria, and Norway.
132	Indigotine	Suspected carcinogen, linked to hyperactivity, nausea, breathing difficulty, skin reactions, blood pressure. Previously banned in Norway.
133	Brilliant Blue	Suspected carcinogen, linked to hyperactivity, asthmatics should avoid. Previously banned in Belgium, France, Germany, Switzerland, Sweden, Austria, and Norway.
140	Chlorophyll	
141	Chlorophyll-copper complex	
142	Green S	Hypersensitivity, allergic reactions, asthmatics should avoid. Previously banned in USA, Sweden, Norway, UK..
143	Fast Green FCF	Can cause bladder tumours.
150	Caramel	Linked to gastro intestinal problems, hypersensitivity. Safety suspect. 150(i) seems safest.
150a	Caramel i (Plain Caramel)	Linked to gastro intestinal problems, hypersensitivity. Safety suspect. 150(i) seems safest.
150b	Caramel ii (Caustic Sulphite Caramel)	Linked to gastro intestinal problems, hypersensitivity. Safety suspect. 150(i) seems safest.
150c	Caramel iii (Ammonia Caramel)	Linked to gastro intestinal problems, hypersensitivity. Safety suspect. 150(i) seems safest.
150d	Caramel iv (Sulphite Ammonia Caramel)	Linked to gastro intestinal problems, hypersensitivity. Safety suspect. 150(i) seems safest.

#	NAME	ADVERSE REACTION
151	Brilliant Black BN or Brilliant Black PN	Linked to bowel disorders, hyperactivity, asthmatics should avoid. Previously banned in US, Denmark, France, Germany, Switzerland, Sweden, Austria, Norway.
153	Carbon Black or vegetable carbon	Suspected carcinogen. Previously banned in US.
155	Brown HT	Suspected carcinogen and mutagen. Linked to asthma, skin irritation. Previously banned in US, Denmark, France, Germany, Switzerland, Sweden, Austria, Norway, Belgium.
160a	Carotene	
160b	Annatto extracts	Hypersensitivity, allergic reactions, skin irritations, linked to behaviour and learning problems. Concerns about toxicity still being evaluated by JECFA yet is still freely used.
160c	Paprika oleoresins	Little info available.
160d	Lycopene	
160e	b-apo-8' carotenal	
160f	b-apo-8' carotenoic acid or methyl ethyl ester	
161a	Flavoxanthin	
161b	Lutein	
161c	Kryptoxanthin	
161d	Rubixanthin	
161e	Violoxanthin	
161f	Rhodoxanthin	
161g	Xanthophylls (Canthaxanthin)	
162	Beet red	Considered safe for use in foods and a much better option than coal tar dyes. Avoid for very young children and infants due to high sodium nitrate content.
163	Anthocyanins or grape skin extract or blackcurrant extract	Asthmatics should avoid.

#	NAME	ADVERSE REACTION
164	Saffron or crocetin or crocin	
170	Calcium Carbonate	
171	Titanium Dioxide	Commonly used now in white foods such as vanilla ice cream. Some concern over long-term safety in relation to reproduction and cancer. Regard with caution. Not recommended for regular consumption.
172	Iron oxide	Possible kidney damage. Suspected neurotoxin. Blindness in dog studies.
173	Aluminium	New to standards, previously not permitted in Australia. Previously banned in other countries.
174	Silver	New to standards, previously not permitted in Australia. Previously banned in other countries.
175	Gold	New to standards, previously not permitted in Australia. Previously banned in other countries.
181	Tannic Acid or tannins	Large doses associated with gastric problems, kidney and liver damage.
200–299		
200	Sorbic acid	Skin irritant, behavioural problems. Asthmatics should avoid.
201	Sodium sorbate	Behavioural problems. Linked to asthma and kidney / liver problems.
202	Potassium sorbate	Possible liver damage, behavioural problems. Linked to asthma. Avoid if kidney or heart problems.
203	Calcium sorbate	Behavioural problems. Linked to Asthma and allergic reactions.
210	Benzoic acid	Hyperactivity, asthmatics should avoid, possible neurological dysfunctions.
211	Sodium benzoate	Hyperactivity, asthmatics should avoid, nettle rash, behavioural problems.
212	Potassium benzoate	Asthmatics should avoid, nettle rash, behavioural problems.
213	Calcium benzoate	Asthmatics should avoid, nettle rash, behavioural problems.
216	Propylparaben or propyl -p-hydroxy-benzoate	Asthmatics should avoid, contact dermatitis, eczema, mouth numbing.

#	NAME	ADVERSE REACTION
218	Methylparaben or methyl-p-hydroxy-benzoate	Allergic reactions possible - skin and mouth.
220	Sulphur dioxide	Asthmatics should avoid, gastric irritation /damage, hyperactivity, behavioural problems, poss mutagen. Can be fatal to asthmatics.
221	Sodium sulphite	Asthmatics should avoid, gastric irritation, nausea, nettle rash and swelling, behavioural problems.
222	Sodium bisulphite	Asthmatics should avoid, gastric irritation, nausea, nettle rash and swelling, behavioural problems.
223	Sodium metabisulphite	Asthmatics should avoid, gastric irritation, nausea, nettle rash and swelling, behavioural problems.
224	Potassium metabisulphite	Asthmatics should avoid, gastric irritation, nausea, nettle rash and swelling, behavioural problems.
225	Potassium sulphite	Asthmatics should avoid, gastric irritation, nausea, nettle rash and swelling, behavioural problems.
228	Potassium bisulphite	Asthmatics should avoid, gastric irritation, nausea, nettle rash and swelling, behavioural problems.
234	Nisin	
235	Natamycin or pimaricin	Can cause nausea, vomiting, diarrhoea and skin irritation.
243	Ethyl lauroyl arginate	New to standards – lttle info available
249	Potassium nitrite	Behavioural problems, asthma, breathing difficulties, headaches, dizziness, possible carcinogen. Prohibited in foods for infants and young children.
250	Sodium nitrite	Hyperactivity, behavioural problems, asthma, headaches, dizziness, possible carcinogen. Prohibited in foods for infants and young children.
251	Sodium nitrate	Hyperactivity, behavioural problems, asthma, headaches, dizziness, possible carcinogen. Prohibited in foods for infants and young children.

#	NAME	ADVERSE REACTION
252	Potassium nitrate	Hyperactivity, behavioural problems, asthma, headaches, dizziness, possible carcinogen, kidney inflammation. Prohibited in foods for infants and young children.
260	Acetic acid,glacial	
261	Potassium acetate or potassium diacetate	Those with kidney or liver problems should avoid.
262	Sodium acetates	
263	Calcium acetate	
264	Ammonium acetate	Nausea, vomiting, concerns about carcinogenicity. Avoid where possible, especially for children.
270	Lactic acid	Safe in foods but avoid for very young babies as may be unable to metabolise.
280	Propionic acid	Behavioural and learning problems, headaches. Asthma.
281	Sodium propionate	Behavioural and learning problems, headaches. Asthma.
282	Calcium propionate	Behavioural and learning problems, skin irritation, headaches, migraine. Asthma.
283	Potassium propionate	Behavioural and learning problems, migraine, headaches. Asthma.
290	Carbon dioxide	Reproductive and neurotoxicity, teratogen, possible links to infertility, on NIH hazards list.
296	Malic acid	Safe in foods but avoid for very young babies. Some reports of allergic reactions in sensitive people.
297	Fumaric acid	
300–399		
300	Ascorbic acid	
301	Sodium ascorbate	
302	Calcium ascorbate	Those susceptible to kidney stones should avoid; otherwise regarded as safe.
303	Potassium ascorbate	
304	Ascorbyl palmitate	

#	NAME	ADVERSE REACTION
306	Tocopherols concentrate, mixed	
307	a-Tocopherol	
308	g-Tocopheral	
309	d-Tocopheral	
310	Propyl gallate	Suspected carcinogen, asthmatics and aspirin sensitive people should avoid, liver damage, skin irritations. Prohibited in food for infants and young children as linked to blood disorder.
311	Octyl gallate	Asthmatics and aspirin sensitive people should avoid, gastric and skin irritations. Prohibited in foods for infants and young children
312	Dodecyl gallate	Asthmatics and aspirin sensitive people should avoid, gastric and skin irritations. Prohibited in foods for infants and young children - caused deaths in animal tests.
315	Erythorbic acid	
316	Sodium erythorbate	Headaches reported by some sensitive people. Generally regarded as safe in foods.
319	Tert-butylhydroquinone	Linked to cancer, birth defects and can cause nausea, vomiting, delirium, collapse, and dermatitis. Dose of 5g is fatal - avoid it.
320	Butylated hydroxyanisole	Serious concerns about carcinogenic and estrogenic effects, asthmatics and aspirin sensitive people should avoid, causes metabolic changes and accumulates in body fat. Banned in Japan in 1958 - not permitted in foods for infants and young children.
321	Butylated hydroxytoluene	Suspected carcinogen, asthmatics and aspirin sensitive people should avoid, skin irritation. Prohibited in foods for infants and young children
322	Lecithin	
325	Sodium lactate	
326	Potassium lactate	
327	Calcium lactate	
328	Ammonium lactate	
329	Magnesium lactate	
330	Citric acid	

#	NAME	ADVERSE REACTION
331	Sodium citrates	
332	Potassium citrates	
333	Calcium citrates	
334	Tartaric acid	
335	Sodium tartrates	
336	Potassium tartrate	Those with kidney impairment should avoid.
337	Potassium sodium tartrate	Those with kidney impairment should avoid. Not recommended for those with heart problems or high blood pressure.
338	Phosphoric acid	Neurotoxicity, eye and skin irritant, large doses can lead to acidosis and hypocalcaemia.
339	Sodium phosphates	
340	Potassium phosphates	
341	Calcium phosphates	
342	Ammonium phosphates	New to standards
343	Magnesium phosphates	
349	Ammonium malate	Unsuitable for infants and young children, skin irritations.
350	Sodium malates	
351	Potassium malates	
352	Calcium malates	
353	Metatartaric acid	
354	Calcium tartrate	New to standards
355	Adipic acid	Severe eye irritant, toxic effect in rat studies including death - avoid it.
357	Potassium adipate	
359	Ammonium adipates	New to standards.
363	Succinic acid	New to standards.
365	Sodium fumarate	
366	Potassium fumarate	
367	Calcium fumarate	
368	Ammonium fumarate	New to standards
380	Ammonium citrate or triammonium citrate	May interfere with liver and pancreas function - more study needed.
381	Ferric ammonium citrate	
385	Calcium disodium EDTA	Muscle cramps, kidney damage, gastro-intestinal problems, banned in some countries.

#	NAME	ADVERSE REACTION
400–499		
400	Alginic acid	
401	Sodium alginate	
402	Potassium alginate	
403	Ammonium alginate	
404	Calcium alginate	
405	Propylene glycol alginate	Allergic reactions common, avoid in pregnancy - more study required.
406	Agar	
407	Carrageenan	Suspected carcinogen, linked to ulcerative colitis, damage to the immune system and concern about excitotoxic effects. Not recommended for children – more work needed. Many reports of IBS like symptoms associated with its regular use. Not recommended for regular consumption.
407a	Processed eucheuma seaweed	As above – some studies show that undegraded carrageenan can be broken down into degraded carrageenan in the gut. Regard with caution.
409	Arabinogalactan or larch gum	Allergic reactions, possible weak carcinogen - more work required.
410	Locust bean gum	Large amounts may cause abdominal pain, diarrhoea.
412	Guar gum	
413	Tragacanth gum	Asthma, skin rashes, gastrointestinal upsets, contact dermatitis.
414	Acacia or gum Arabic	Asthma, skin rashes in sensitive people.
415	Xanthan gum	
416	Karaya gum	Asthma. Urticaria, gastrointestinal upsets, dermatitis.
417	Tara gum	New to standrds – little info available ·
418	Gellan gum	
420	Sorbitol or sorbitol syrup	Not suitable for diabetics, infants and young children, liver toxicity, gastrointestinal upsets. Prohibited in foods for infants and young children.
421	Mannitol	Not for diabetics, infants and young children, or those with kidney / liver impairment. Linked to hyperactivity, kidney damage. On NIH Hazards list.
422	Glycerin or glycerol	Headaches, high blood sugar levels, eye skin irritation in sensitive people.

#	NAME	ADVERSE REACTION
431	Polyethylene (40) stearate	Suspected carcinogen, skin allergies - new to standard.
432	Polysorbate 20 or polyoxyethylene sorbitan monolaurate	Suspected carcinogen - more work needed.
433	Polysorbate 80 or polyoxyethylene (20) sorbitan monooleate	Suspected carcinogen - more work needed.
435	Polysorbate 60	Suspected carcinogen - more testing needed.
436	Polysorbate 65	Suspected carcinogen - more testing needed.
440	Pectins	
440a	Pectins	
440b	Pectins	
441	Gelatine	
442	Ammonium salts of phosphatidic acid	
444	Sucrose acetate isobutyrate	
445	Gylcerol esters of wood rosins	Headaches, high blood sugar levels, eye skin irritation in sensitive people.
450	Potassium pyrophosphate (also listed as sodium acid pyrophosphate and sodium pyrophosphate)	Linked to kidney stones in susceptible people, otherwise regarded as safe.
451	Potassium tripolyphosphate (also listed as sodium tripolyphosphate)	Linked to kidney stones in susceptible people, otherwise regarded as safe.
452	Potassium polymetaphosphate (also listed as sodium metaphosphate insoluble and sodium polyphosphates glassy)	Linked to kidney stones in susceptible people, otherwise regarded as safe.
460	Cellulose microcrystalline and powdered	Most sources regard as safe although banned in UK in baby food only.
461	Methyl cellulose	

#	NAME	ADVERSE REACTION
463	Hydroxypropyl cellulose	
464	Hydroxypropyl methylcellulose	
465	Methyl ethyl cellulose	Flatulence, intestinal upsets, diarrhoea.
466	Sodium carboxymethylcellulose	Suspected carcinogen, flatulence, intestinal discomfort and diarrhoea.
470	Aluminuim, calcium, sodium, magnesium, potassium and ammonium salts of fatty acids.	
471	Mono and di glycerides of fatty acids	
472a	Acetic and fatty acid esters of glycerol	
472b	Lactic and fatty acid esters of glycerol	
472c	Citric and fatty acid esters of glycerol	
472e	Diacetyltartaric and fatty acid esters of glycerol	Headaches, high blood sugar levels, eye skin irritation in sensitive people. JECFA still evaluating.
472f	Mixed tartaric acetic and fatty acid esters of glycerol	
473	Sucrose esters of fatty acids	
475	Polyglycerol esters of fatty acids	
476	Polyglycerol esters of interesterified ricinoleic acid	
477	Propylene glycol mono and di-esters	Derived from propylene glycol.
480	Dioctyl sodium sulphosuccinate	More testing being done especially in relation to children and infants.
481	Sodium lactylate	
482	Calcium lactylate (also listed as calcium oleyl lactylate and calcium stearoyl lactylate)	Adverse reactions have occurred in animal tests.

#	NAME	ADVERSE REACTION
491	Sorbitan monostearate	Some adverse effects recorded in animal studies in large doses – growth retardation. Considered safe in foods in low doses – more studies needed.
492	Sorbitan tristearate	Some adverse effects recorded in animal studies in large doses – growth retardation. Considered safe in foods in low doses – more studies needed.
500–599		
500	Sodium carbonate or bi carbonate	Regarded as safe in small amounts.
501	Potassium carbonates	
503	Ammonium bicarbonate or ammonium hydrogen carbonate	Can irritate mucous membranes and lead to skin and scalp irritations in some people.
504	Magnesium carbonate	
507	Hydrochloric acid	Stomach and mouth irritant - some sources list as possible teratogenic.
508	Potassium chloride	Associated with gastric ulcers, circulatory collapse, nausea, and liver toxicity. Not recommended for children.
509	Calcium chloride	Stomach irritant in sensitive people.
510	Ammonium chloride	Large amounts can cause acidosis - nausea, headaches, and insomnia. Those with kidney / liver problems should avoid.
511	Magnesium chloride	Caused kidney damage in dogs so those with kidney damage may wish to avoid.
512	Stannous chloride	Nausea, headache, gastric upset. Skin and mucous membrane irritant.
514	Sodium sulphate	Unsuitable for infants and children and those with kidney /liver problems due to high sodium content - Skin irritant.
515	Potassium sulphate	Regarded as safe in small doses.
516	Calcium sulphate	
518	Magnesium sulphate	Laxative effect, low blood pressure, drowsiness, those with kidney damage should avoid.
519	Cupric sulphate	Linked to gastrointestinal problems, those with kidney / liver problems should avoid, neurotoxicity.

#	NAME	ADVERSE REACTION
526	Calcium hydroxide	
529	Calcium oxide	
530	Magnesium oxide	Caused tumours in hamsters - can cause diarrhoea.
535	Sodium ferrocyanide	
536	Potassium ferrocyanide	
541	Sodium aluminium phosphate	Thought to release aluminium during digestion - concerns about skeletal abnormalities, dementia, and Parkinson's type illness.
542	Bone phosphate	
551	Silicon dioxide	
552	Calcium silicate	
553	Magnesium silicate or talc	Linked to stomach and ovarian cancers. Respiratory problems.
554	Sodium aluminosilicate	Linked to Alzheimer's and nerve damage, bone diseases, kidney damage, and neurotoxicity.
555	Potassium aluminium silicate	Linked to Alzheimer's and nerve damage, bone diseases, kidney damage, and neurotoxicity.
556	Calcium aluminium silicate	Linked to Alzheimer's and nerve damage, bone diseases, kidney damage, and neurotoxicity.
558	Bentonite	
559	Aluminium silicate	
560	Potassium silicate	Little info available.
570	Stearic acid or fatty acid	Can cause allergic reactions in sensitive people - skin irritant.
575	Glucono d-lactone or glucono delta lactone	
577	Potassium gluconate	
578	Calcium gluconate	
579	Ferrous gluconate	Diarrhoea, vomiting, gastrointestinal upsets. Research showed it caused tumours in mice. Regard with caution.

#	NAME	ADVERSE REACTION
580	Magnesium gluconate	New to standards - no info avail - regard with caution.
586	4-Hexylresorcinol	New to standards - no info avail - regard with caution.
600–899		
620	L-Glutamic acid	Unsuitable for infants and children, allergic and hypersensitive reactions, headaches, nausea, sleeplessness.
621	Monosodium L-glutamate or MSG	Asthma, hyperactivity, depression, mood changes, sleeplessness, nausea, migraine, linked to infertility, teratogen, convulsions, abdominal discomfort. See text re other hidden sources of MSG.
622	Monopotassium L-glutamate	Problems in people with poor kidney function, headache, asthma, nausea, restlessness.
623	Calcium glutamate	Asthmatics and aspirin sensitive people should avoid.
624	Monoammonium L-glutamate	Varied allergic reactions in some people. Not recommended for asthmatics.
625	Magnesium glutamate	Varied allergic reactions in some people. Not recommended for asthmatics.
627	Disodium 5'-guanylate	Asthmatics and aspirin sensitive people should avoid, linked to hyperactivity, gout sufferers avoid. Prohibited in foods for infants and young children.
631	Disodium 5'-inosinate	May trigger gout symptoms, varied reactions reported. Prohibited in foods for infants and young children. Not recommended for asthmatics.
635	Disodium 5'-ribonucleotides	Can cause terrible itchy skin rashes, hyperactivity, sleeplessness, mood changes, many varied ill effects reported. Previously banned in some other countries -very common in Aust foods. Asthmatics should avoid.
636	Maltol	More work needed – regard with caution.
637	Ethyl maltol	Some concerns about toxicity- more work required.

#	NAME	ADVERSE REACTION
640	Glycine	Some concerns about long-term safety – more study needed as use becomes more widespread.
641	L-Leucine	Caused birth defects in laboratory animals - more testing needed - Regard with caution.
900–1099		
900a	Polydimethylsiloxane or dimethylpolysiloxane	Suspected carcinogen. Can contain formaldehyde.
901	Beeswax white and yellow	Occasionally causes allergic reactions in sensitive people.
903	Carnauba wax	Rare skin allergy reported in sensitive people.
904	Shellac	Rare skin allergy in sensitive people
905b	Petrolatum or Petroleum jelly	Can inhibit absorption of digestive fats, allergic skin reactions possible in some people.
914	Oxidised polyethylene	Linked to cancer, kidney and liver damage. Used as a protective coating on fruits, nuts and vegetables.
920	L-Cysteine monohydrochloride	Derived from human hair – commonly used in bread products.
941	Nitrogen	
942	Nitrous oxide	
943a	Butane	Caused cancer in animal tests, neurotoxicity, on NIH Hazards list. Petroleum derivative - avoid it.
943b	Isobutane	Neurotoxic at high concentrations; on NIH hazards list.
944	Propane	Neurotoxic at high concentrations; on NIH hazards list.
946	Octafluorocyclobutane	More info needed - regard with caution.
950	Acesulphame potassium	Caused cancer and tumours in animal tests.
951	Aspartame	Linked to many health problems including cancer, asthma, nausea, depressions, hyperactivity, and seizures. The most complained about food additive accounting for 75% of all complaints to FDA.

#	NAME	ADVERSE REACTION
952	Calcium cyclamate or sodium cyclamate	Suspected carcinogen, animal tests caused testicular damage and embryo damage in rats. Previously banned in UK and USA in 1970 but still permitted in Australia.
953	Isomalt	
954	Saccharin or calcium / sodium / potassium saccharin	Known carcinogen especially linked to bladder and reproductive cancers. Previously banned in US in 1977 but reinstated with strict labelling provisions.
955	Sucralose	Linked to neurological and immunological disorders, caused kidney and liver damage in tests. More research needed - avoid it.
956	Alitame	Liver abnormalities in lab tests - more research needed.
957	Thaumatin	Not for use in infants' foods. Little information available - regard with caution.
961	Neotame	Little info available – similar to aspartame so regard with caution.
960	Steviol gycosides	Recently added to standards – currently regarded as safe.
962	Aspartame – acesulphame salt	New to standards – little info available. Similar to aspartame so regard with caution.
965	Maltitol and maltitol syrup or hydrogenated glucose syrup	Caused increased incidence of tumours in animal tests.
966	Lactitol	Diarrhoea in high doses, more work needed.
967	Xylitol	Diarrhoea, stomach upsets, early studies showed carcinogenic potential. More recently regarded as safe in small doses. More work needed.
968	Erythritol	Little info available - regard with caution.
999 (i)	Quillaia extract (type 1)	New to standards – little info available
999 (ii)	Quillaia exract (type 2)	New to standards – little info available
1001	Choline salts	New to standards – little info available

#	NAME	ADVERSE REACTION
1100–		
1100	a-amylase	
1101	Proteases (papain, bromelain, ficin)	Little info available.
1102	Glucose oxidase	Little info available.
1104	Lipases	
1105	Lysozyme	
1200	Polydextrose	
1201	Polyvinylpyrrolidone	Cancer, lung and kidney damage; liver toxicity, allergic reactions, skin reactions. Made from acetylene, hydrogen, formaldehyde, ammonia
1400	Dextrin roasted starch	Allergic reactions reported, celiacs should avoid
1401	Acid treated starch	Allergic reactions reported, celiacs should avoid
1402	Alkaline treated starch	Allergic reactions reported, celiacs should avoid
1403	Bleached starch	Linked to asthma as may be treated with sulphur dioxide
1404	Oxidised starch	Linked to asthma as may be treated with sulphur dioxide
1405	Enzyme treated starch	Allergic reactions reported, celiacs should avoid
1410	Monostarch phosphate	
1412	Distarch phosphate	
1413	Phosphated distarch phosphate	
1414	Acetylated distarch phosphate	
1420	Starch acetate esterified with acetic anhydride	Allergic reactions reported, celiacs should avoid
1422	Acetylated distarch adipate	Animal tests showed slowed growth rates and renal lesions. Common in baby foods.
1440	Hydroxypropyl starch	

#	NAME	ADVERSE REACTION
1442	Hydroxypropyl distarch phosphate	
1450	Starch sodium octenylsuccinate	
1505	Triethyl citrate	
1518	Triacetin	
1520	Propylene glycol	Large doses can be toxic, kidney failure, depression of CNS, liver damage, teratogen, on NIH Hazards list. Humectant used to coat fruit and vegetables. USA has placed a total recall of any medication containing this additive yet still permitted in food.
1521	Polyethylene glycol 8000	Caused renal failure in some tests, more info needed, avoid it for now
1522	Calcium lignosulphonate (40 – 60)	New to standards – little info available

Appendix 5: Food Additives Alphabetical Listing

PRESCRIBED NAME	NUMBER

Symbols used in this list:

a = alpha; *b* = beta; *d* = delta; *g* = gamma.

Prescribed Name	Code Number
Acacia or gum Arabic (thickener, stabiliser)	414
Acesulphame potassium (sweetener)	950
Acetic acid, glacial (acidity regulator)	260
Acetic and fatty acid esters of glycerol (emulsifier, stabiliser)	472a
Acetylated distarch adipate (thickener, stabiliser)	1422
Acetylated distarch phosphate (thickener, stabiliser)	1414
Acid treated starch (thickener, stabiliser)	1401
Adipic acid (acidity regulator)	355
Advantame (sweetener)	
Agar (thickener, gelling agent, stabiliser)	406
Alginic acid (thickener, stabiliser)	400
Alitame (sweetener)	956
Alkaline treated starch (thickener, stabiliser)	1402
Alkanet or Alkannin (colour)	103
Allura red AC (colour)	129
Aluminium (colour)	173
Aluminium, calcium, sodium, magnesium, potassium and ammonium salts of fatty acids (emulsifier, stabiliser, anti-caking agent)	470
Aluminium silicate	559

Amaranth (colour)	123
Ammonium acetate (acidity regulator)	264
Ammonium adipates (acidity regulator)	359
Ammonium alginate (thickener, stabiliser)	403
Ammonium bicarbonate or Ammonium hydrogen carbonate (acidity regulator, raising agent)	503
Ammonium chloride (bulking agent)	510
Ammonium citrate or triammonium citrate (acidity regulator)	380
Ammonium fumarate (acidity regulator)	368
Ammonium lactate (acidity regulator)	328
Ammonium malate (acidity regulator)	349
Ammonium phosphates (acidity regulator)	342
Ammonium salts of phosphatidic acid (emulsifier)	442
alpha - amylase (enzyme)	1100
Annatto extracts (colour)	160b
Anthocyanins or Grape skin extract or Blackcurrant extract (colour)	163
Arabinogalactan or Larch gum (thickener, gelling agent, stabiliser)	409
Ascorbic acid (antioxidant)	300
Ascorbyl palmitate (antioxidant)	304
Aspartame (sweetener)	951
Aspartame – acesulphame salt (sweetener)	962
Azorubine or Carmoisine (colour)	122
beta-apo-8' Carotenal (colour)	160e
beta-apo-8' Carotenoic acid methyl or ethyl ester (colour)	160f
Beeswax, white and yellow (glazing agent)	901
Beet red (colour)	162
Bentonite (anti-caking agent)	558
Benzoic acid (preservative)	210
Bleached starch (thickener, stabiliser)	1403

Bone phosphate (anti-caking agent, emulsifier)	542
Brilliant black BN or Brilliant black PN (colour)	151
Brilliant blue FCF (colour)	133
Brown HT (colour)	155
Butane (propellant)	943a
Butylated hydroxyanisole (antioxidant)	320
Butylated hydroxytoluene (antioxidant)	321
Calcium acetate (acidity regulator)	263
Calcium alginate (thickener, stabiliser, gelling agent)	404
Calcium aluminium silicate (anti-caking agent)	556
Calcium ascorbate (antioxidant)	302
Calcium benzoate (preservative)	213
Calcium carbonate (colour, anti-caking agent)	170
Calcium chloride (firming agent)	509
Calcium citrates (acidity regulator, stabiliser)	333
Calcium cyclamate or sodium cyclamate or cyclamate (sweetener)	952
Calcium disodium ethylenediaminetetraacetate or calcium disodium EDTA (preservative, antioxidant)	385
Calcium fumarate (acidity regulator)	367
Calcium gluconate (acidity regulator, firming agent)	578
Calcium glutamate (flavour enhancer)	623
Calcium hydroxide (acidity regulator, firming agent)	526
Calcium lactate (acidity regulator)	327
Calcium lactylate or Calcium oleyl lactylate or Calcium stearoyl lactylate (emulsifier, stabiliser)	482
Calcium malates (acidity regulator)	352
Calcium oxide (acidity regulator)	529
Calcium phosphates (acidity regulator, emulsifier, stabiliser, anti-caking agent)	341

Calcium propionate (preservative)	282
Calcium silicate (anti-caking agent)	552
Calcium sorbate (preservative)	203
Calcium sulphate (firming agent)	516
Calcium tartrate (acidity regulator)	354
Caramel I (colour)	150a
Caramel II (colour)	150b
Caramel III (colour)	150c
Caramel IV (colour)	150d
Carbon black or vegetable carbon (colour)	153
Carbon dioxide (propellant)	290
Carmines or Carminic acid or Cochineal (colour)	120
Carnauba wax (glazing agent)	903
Carotene (colour)	160a
Carrageenan (thickener, gelling agent, stabiliser)	407
Cellulose microcrystalline and powdered (anti-caking agent)	460
Chlorophyll (colour)	140
Chlorophyll-copper complex (colour)	141
Choline salts (emulsifier)	1001
Citric acid (acidity regulator, antioxidant)	330
Citric and fatty acid esters of glycerol (emulsifier, stabiliser)	472c
Cupric sulphate (mineral salt)	519
Curcumin or Turmeric (colour)	100
Dextrin roasted starch (thickener, stabiliser)	1400
Diacetyltartaric and fatty acid esters of glycerol (emulsifier)	472e
Dimethyl dicarbonate (preservative)	242
Dioctyl sodium sulphosuccinate (emulsifier)	480
Disodium 5 -guanylate (flavour enhancer)	627
Disodium 5 -inosinate (flavour enhancer)	631

Disodium 5'-ribonucleotides (flavour enhancer)	635
Distarch phosphate (thickener, stabiliser)	1412
Dodecyl gallate (antioxidant)	312
Ethyl lauroyl arginate (preservative)	243
Ethyl maltol (flavour enhancer)	637
Enzyme treated starches (thickener, stabiliser)	1405
Erythorbic acid (antioxidant)	315
Erythritol (humectant, sweetener)	968
Erythrosine (colour)	127
Fast green FCF (colour)	143
Ferric ammonium citrate (acidity regulator, anti-caking agent)	381
Ferrous gluconate (colour retention agent)	579
Flavoxanthin (colour)	161a
Fumaric acid (acidity regulator)	297
Gellan gum (thickener, stabiliser, gelling agent)	418
Glucono *delta* -lactone or Glucono delta-lactone (acidity regulator, raising agent)	575
Glucose oxidase (antioxidant)	1102
Glycerin or glycerol (humectant)	422
Glycerol esters of wood rosins (emulsifier, stabiliser)	445
Glycine (flavour enhancer)	640
Gold (colour)	175
Green S (colour)	142
Guar gum (thickener, stabiliser)	412
4-Hexylresorcinol (antioxidant)	586
Hydrochloric acid (acidity regulator)	507
Hydroxypropyl cellulose (thickener, stabiliser, emulsifier)	463
Hydroxypropyl distarch phosphate (thickener, stabiliser)	1442
Hydroxypropyl methylcellulose (thickener, stabiliser, emulsifier)	464

Hydroxypropyl starch (thickener, stabiliser)	1440
Indigotine (colour)	132
Iron oxide (colour)	172
Isobutane (propellant)	943b
Isomalt (humectant, sweetener, bulking agent, anti-caking agent)	953
Karaya gum (thickener, stabiliser)	416
Kryptoxanthin (colour)	161c
Lactic acid (acidity regulator)	270
Lactic and fatty acid esters of glycerol (emulsifier, stabiliser)	472b
Lactitol (sweetener, humectant)	966
L-Cysteine monohydrochloride (raising agent)	920
Lecithin (antioxidant, emulsifier)	322
L-Glutamic acid (flavour enhancer)	620
Lipases (enzyme)	1104
L-Leucine (flavour enhancer)	641
Locust bean gum or Carob bean gum (thickener, stabiliser)	410
Lutein (colour)	161b
Lycopene (colour)	160d
Lysozyme (enzyme, preservative)	1105
Magnesium carbonate (acidity regulator, anti-caking agent)	504
Magnesium chloride (firming agent)	511
Magnesium gluconate (acidity regulatory, firming agent)	580
Magnesium glutamate (flavour enhancer)	625
Magnesium lactate (acidity regulator)	329
Magnesium oxide (anti-caking agent)	530
Magnesium phosphates (acidity regulator, anti-caking agent)	343
Magnesium silicate or Talc (anti-caking agent)	553
Magnesium sulphate (firming agent)	518
Malic acid (acidity regulator)	296

Maltitol and maltitol syrup or hydrogenated glucose syrup (sweetener, stabiliser, emulsifier, humectant)	965
Maltol (flavour enhancer)	636
Mannitol (sweetener, humectant)	421
Metatartaric acid (acidity regulator)	353
Methyl ethyl cellulose (thickener, stabiliser, emulsifier, foaming agent)	465
Methyl cellulose (thickener, stabiliser, emulsifier)	461
Methylparaben or Methyl-p-hydroxy-benzoate (preservative)	218
Mixed tartaric, acetic and fatty acid esters of glycerol (emulsifier, stabiliser)	472f
Mono- and di-glycerides of fatty acids (emulsifier, stabiliser)	471
Monoammonium L-glutamate (flavour enhancer)	624
Monopotassium L-glutamate (flavour enhancer)	622
Monosodium L-glutamate or MSG (flavour enhancer)	621
Monostarch phosphate (thickener, stabiliser)	1410
Natamycin or Pimaricin (preservative)	235
Neotame (sweetener)	961
Nisin (preservative)	234
Nitrogen (propellant)	941
Nitrous oxide (propellant)	942
Octafluorocyclobutane (propellant)	946
Octyl gallate (antioxidant)	311
Oxidised polyethylene (humectant)	914
Oxidised starch (thickener, stabiliser)	1404
Paprika oleoresins (colour)	160c
Pectins (thickener, stabiliser, gelling agent)	440
Petrolatum or petroleum jelly (glazing agent)	905b
Phosphated distarch phosphate (thickener, stabiliser)	1413
Phosphoric acid (acidity regulator)	338

Polydextrose (humectant, bulking agent, stabiliser, thickener)	1200
Polydimethylsiloxane or Dimethylpolysiloxane (anti-caking agent, emulsifier)	900a
Polyethylene (40) stearate (emulsifier)	431
Polyethylene glycol 8000 (antifoaming agent)	1521
Polyglycerol esters of fatty acids (emulsifier)	475
Polyglycerol esters of interesterified ricinoleic acid (emulsifier)	476
Polysorbate 60 or Polyoxyethylene (20) sorbitan monostearate (emulsifier)	435
Polysorbate 65 or Polyoxyethylene (20) sorbitan tristearate (emulsifier)	436
Polysorbate 80 or Polyoxyethylene (20) sorbitan monooleate (emulsifier)	433
Polyvinylpyrrolidone (stabiliser)	1201
Ponceau 4R (colour)	124
Potassium acetate or Potassium diacetate (acidity regulator)	261
Potassium adipate (acidity regulator)	357
Potassium alginate (thickener, stabiliser)	402
Potassium aluminium silicate	555
Potassium ascorbate (antioxidant)	303
Potassium benzoate (preservative)	212
Potassium bisulphite (preservative)	228
Potassium carbonates (acidity regulator, stabiliser)	501
Potassium chloride (gelling agent)	508
Potassium citrates (acidity regulator, stabiliser)	332
Potassium ferrocyanide (anti-caking agent)	536
Potassium fumarate (acidity regulator)	366
Potassium gluconate (sequestrant)	577
Potassium lactate (acidity regulator, humectant, bulking agent)	326
Potassium malates (acidity regulator)	351
Potassium metabisulphite (preservative)	224
Potassium nitrate (preservative, colour fixative)	252

Potassium nitrite (preservative, colour fixative)	249
Potassium phosphates (acidity regulator, emulsifier, stabiliser)	340
Potassium polymetaphosphate or Sodium metaphosphate, insoluble or Sodium polyphosphates, glassy (emulsifier, stabiliser)	452
Potassium propionate (preservative)	283
Potassium pyrophosphate or Sodium acid pyrophosphate or Sodium pyrophosphate (emulsifiers, acidity regulators, stabilisers)	450
Potassium silicate (anti-caking agent)	560
Potassium sodium tartrate (acidity regulator, stabiliser)	337
Potassium sorbate (preservative)	202
Potassium sulphate (acidity regulator)	515
Potassium sulphite (preservative)	225
Potassium tartrate or Potassium acid tartrate (acidity regulator, stabiliser)	336
Potassium tripolyphosphate or Sodium tripolyphosphate (acidity regulator)	451
Processed eucheuma seaweed (thickener, gelling agent, stabiliser)	407a
Propane (propellant)	944
Propionic acid (preservative)	280
Propyl gallate (antioxidant)	310
Propylene glycol (humectant)	1520
Propylene glycol alginate (thickener, emulsifier)	405
Propylene glycol mono- and di-esters or Propylene glycol esters of fatty acids (emulsifier)	477
Propylparaben or Propyl-p-hydroxy-benzoate (preservative)	216
Proteases (papain, bromelain, ficin) (stabiliser, enzyme)	1101
Quillaia extract (type 1) (emulsifier)	999(i)
Quilaia extract (type 2) (emulsifier)	999(ii)
Quinoline yellow (colour)	104
Rhodoxanthin (colour)	161f
Riboflavin or Riboflavin 5'-phosphate sodium (colour)	101

Rubixanthin (colour)	161d
Saccharin or calcium saccharin or sodium saccharine or potassium saccharine (sweetener)	954
Saffron or Crocetin or Crocin (colour)	164
Shellac (glazing agent)	904
Silicon dioxide, amorphous (anti-caking agent)	551
Silver (colour)	174
Sodium acetates (acidity regulator)	262
Sodium acid pyrophosphate (leavening agent, stabiliser)	450
Sodium alginate (thickener, stabiliser, gelling agent)	401
Sodium aluminium phosphate (acidity regulator, emulsifier)	541
Sodium aluminosilicate (anti-caking agent)	554
Sodium ascorbate (antioxidant)	301
Sodium benzoate (preservative)	211
Sodium bisulphite (preservative)	222
Sodium carbonate or Sodium bicarbonate (acidity regulator, raising agent, anti-caking agent)	500
Sodium carboxymethylcellulose (thickener, stabiliser)	466
Sodium citrates (acidity regulator, emulsifier, stabiliser)	331
Sodium erythorbate (antioxidant)	316
Sodium ferrocyanide (anti-caking agent)	535
Sodium fumarate (acidity regulator)	365
Sodium lactate (acidity regulator, humectant, bulking agent)	325
Sodium lactylate or sodium oleyl lactylate or sodium stearoyl lactylate (emulsifier, stabiliser)	481
Sodium malates (acidity regulator, humectant)	350
Sodium metabisulphite (preservative)	223
Sodium metaphosphate, insoluble (Emulsifier)	452
Sodium nitrate (preservative, colour fixative)	251
Sodium nitrite (preservative, colour fixative)	250

Sodium phosphates (acidity regulator, emulsifier, stabiliser)	339
Sodium polyphosphates, glassy (emulsifier)	452
Sodium propionate (preservative)	281
Sodium pyrophosphate (leavening agent stabiliser)	450
Sodium sorbate (preservative)	201
Sodium sulphate (acidity regulator)	514
Sodium sulphite (preservative)	221
Sodium tartrates (acidity regulator)	335
Sodium tripolyphosphate (leavening agent,stabiliser)	451
Sorbic acid (preservative)	200
Sorbitan monostearate (emulsifier)	491
Sorbitan tristearate (emulsifier)	492
Sorbitol or sorbitol syrup (sweetener, humectant, emulsifier)	420
Stannous chloride (antioxidant)	512
Starch acetate esterified with acetic anhydride (thickener, stabiliser)	1420
Starch sodium octenylsuccinate (thickener, stabiliser)	1450
Stearic acid or fatty acid (glazing agent, foaming agent)	570
Steviol gycosides (sweetener)	960
Succinic acid (acidity regulator)	363
Sucralose (sweetener)	955
Sucrose acetate isobutyrate (emulsifier, stabiliser)	444
Sucrose esters of fatty acids (emulsifier)	473
Sulphur dioxide (preservative)	220
Sunset yellow FCF (colour)	110
Tannic acid or tannins (colour, emulsifier, stabiliser, thickener)	181
Tara Gum (thickener / stabiliser)	417
Tartaric acid (acidity regulator, antioxidant)	334
Tartrazine (colour)	102
tert-Butylhydroquinone (antioxidant)	319
Thaumatin (flavour enhancer, sweetener)	957

Titanium dioxide (colour)	171
alpha -Tocopherol (antioxidant)	307
delta -Tocopherol (antioxidant)	309
gamma -Tocopherol (antioxidant)	308
Tocopherols concentrate, mixed (antioxidant)	306
Tragacanth gum (thickener, stabiliser)	413
Triacetin (humectant)	1518
Triethyl citrate (antifoaming agent)	1505
Violoxanthin (colour)	161e
Xanthan gum (thickener, stabiliser)	415
Xylitol (sweetener, humectant, stabiliser)	967

References

The author gratefully acknowledges the following sources of reference used in researching and compiling this book. Whilst every attempt has been made to trace and acknowledge copyright of all sources, if any sources have not been acknowledged, Additive Alert would be pleased to hear from the copyright owners so any omission can be rectified.

Books

Borushek Allan; *Allan Borushek's Pocket Calorie and Fat Counter*; Family Health Publications, WA Australia 2002

Buist Robert; *Food Sensitivity*; Harper and Row Publishers, NSW Australia 1986

Davis Damien; *Are You Poisoning Your Family*; Lamont Publishing, VIC Australia 1992

Dengate Sue; *Fed Up With Asthma*; Random House Australia, NSW Australia 2003

Dengate Sue; *Fed Up;* Random House Australia, NSW Australia 1998

Dingle Peter, Brown Toni; *Cosmetics and Personal Care Dangerous Beauty*; 1999

Dingle Peter, Brown Toni; *Sick Homes Part 1: Volatile Chemicals*; 1999

Dingle Peter; *The DEAL for Happier, Healthier, Smarter Kids*; 2004

Epstein Samuel S; *Unreasonable Risk*; Environmental Toxicology, Illinois USA 2002

Fisher Jo; *Food for Thought*; Heinemann Library 1997

Food Standards Australia New Zealand; *Food Additives and Labels*; Murdoch Books, NSW Australia 2002

FSANZ, *Benzene in flavoured Beverages*; June 2006

Hanssen Maurice; *The New Additive Code Breaker*; Lothian Books, VIC Australia 1989

Hermanussen and others, *Obesity, voracity and short stature: the impact of glutamate on the regulation of appetite*, Eur J Clii Nutr 2005

Jeffreys Toni Ph.D; *Your Health At Risk;* Thorsons; 1999

Lau K and others, *Synergistic Interactions between Commonly used Food Additives in a Developmental Neurotoxicity Test*, Toxicol Sci 2005 Dec 13

Millstone Eric, Abraham John; *ADDITIVES A Guide for Everyone;* Penquin Books, London 1988

Pleshette Janet; *Health On Your Plate*; Arrow Books, London 1983

Simontacchi Carol; *The Crazy Makers: How the Food Industry is Destroying Our Brains and Harming Our Children*; Penquin Putnam Inc, New York USA 2000

Statham Bill; *The Chemical Maze 2nd Edition*; POSSIBILITY. COM, VIC Australia 2002

Treffers Sue; *Food Additives Pocket Reference Series*; Mastercorp Pty Ltd, QLD Australia 2003

Internet sources

About Asthma; Asthma Australia;
    www.asthmaaustralia.org.au/asthma

ADD and Diet; A Current Affair Factsheet 25 April 2000;
    www.ninemsn.com.au

Chemical Cuisine CSPI's Guide to Food Additives; Centre for
    Science in the Public Interest;
    www.cspinet.orgreports/chemcuisine

*Chemicals combine in our bodies but are rarely tested that
    way. Why?;* Centre for Children's Health and the
    Environment, Mount Sinai School of Medicine;
    www.childenvironment.org

Do Food Additives Subtract from Health?; Business Week;
    www.businessweek.com/1996

Food Additives Guide; www.foodag.com

*Food Additives- What you always wanted to know about food
    additives but had no one to ask*; Food Allergy Centre;
    www.x-sitez.com/allergy/additives

Food Additives: Are they making us sick?; A Current Affair
    Factsheet 17 January 2002; www.ninemsn.com.au

Food Additives: Common Types; A Current Affair Factsheet
    17 January 2002; www.ninemsn.com.au

Food Additives; BBC News 6 October 1999 Health Medical
    Notes; www.news.bbc.co.uk

Food Additives; Food Standards Australia New Zealand;
    www.foodstandards.gov.au

Food Additives; Nutrition Australia;
    www.nutritionaustralia.org/Food_Facts/FAQ

References

Food Additives–detailed list of effects; Quackbusters;
www.quackbusters.com.au/food_additives

Food Allergy or Food Intolerance?; Food Intolerance Network
Factsheet; www.fedupwithfoodadditives.info/factsheets

Food: Food Safety Food Additives; Choice;
www.choice.au/articles

Gold Mark D; *Monosodium Glutamate (MSG)*;
www.holisticmed.com/msg

Gold Mark D; *The Bitter Truth About Artificial Sweeteners*;
Extracted from Nexus Magazine Volume 2/ 28 and
Volume 3/1; www.nexusmagazine.com/Aspartame

Goodspeed Michael; *Processed Foods May Damage the
Developing Brain*; 1999; www.rense.com/health3

Guide to Food Additives; Food Allergy Centre;
www.x-sitez.com/allergy/additives

Haas Elson MD; *Food Additives and Human Health*;
Extract from Staying Healthy Shopper's Guide:
Feed Your Family Safely; Healthy Child online;
www.healthychild.com

*Johnny can't read, sit still or stop hitting the neighbour's
kid. Why?;* Centre for Children's Health and the
Environment, Mount Sinai School of Medicine;
www.childenvironment.org

List of substances scheduled for evaluation or re-evaluation;
Joint FAO/WHO Expert Committee on Food Additives
(JECFA) Sixty First meeting Rome, 10–19 June 2003;
www.x-sitez.com/allergy/additives/vege400-495

More Kids Are Getting Brain Cancer. Why?; Centre for
Children's Health and the Environment, Mount Sinai
School of Medicine; www.childenvironment.org

Our most precious natural resource is being threatened. Why?;
Centre for Children's Health and the Environment,
Mount Sinai School of Medicine;
www.childenvironment.org

Pesticides could become the ultimate male contraceptive. Why?;
Centre for Children's Health and the Environment,
Mount Sinai School of Medicine;
www.childenvironment.org

Schardt David; *Diet and Behaviour in Children*; Nutrition
Action Newsletter March 2000; www.cspinet.org/nah

She's the test subject for thousands of toxic chemicals. Why?;
Centre for Children's Health and the Environment,
Mount Sinai School of Medicine;
www.childenvironment.org

Splenda Information Sheet; Sucralose Toxicity Information
Centre; www.holisticmed.com/splenda

The Bread Preservative (282); Food Intolerance Network
Factsheet; www.fedupwithfoodadditives.info/factsheets

The Hyperactive Children's Support Group; www.hacsg.org.uk

Trouble may begin in the grocery cart; Feingold Association of
the United States; www.feingold.org

Press and media articles

Arma Ingrid; *My sandwich is toxic*; The Sunday Times,
8 September 2002

Asthma fight stepped up; The West Australian, 26 August 2002

Dalton Rodney; *Waistline deadline*; The Weekend Australian,
22 June 2002

Frozen fat the choice in chips; The West Australian,
9 September 2003

References

Healthy Scepticism; The Weekend Australian, 5 July 2003

James Amanda; *WA Top state for 'dexies'*; The West
    Australian, 4 September 2002

James Amanda; *WA youth taller but much fatter*; The West
    Australian, 11 September 2002

Laurie Victoria; *A battle plan to save the children of a 'toxic
    society'*; The Australian, 2002

Laurie Victoria; *The Hyper State*; The Weekend Australian
    Magazine, 8 February 2003

McKimmie Marnie; *Depression food link raised*; The West
    Australian, 11 February 2004

Milburn Caroline; *Children in crisis: expert*; The West
    Australian, 9 November 2002

Miller Margaret; *Busy teens grab junk food*; The West
    Australian, 25 June 2003

O'Leary Cathy; *Asthma record among the worst;* The West
    Australian, 6 May 2004

O'Leary Cathy; *Diabetes alert for obese children*; The West
    Australian, 5 May 2004

O'Leary Cathy; *New wave of young diabetics*; The West
    Australian, 25 November 2003

O'Leary Cathy; *Not so sweet findings for additive*; The West
    Australian, 10 May 2004

Pemble Lousie; *Forget the gimmicks and go back to basics*;
    The Weekend Australian, 5 July 2003

Rasdien Peta; *Warnings on high-fat food wanted: survey*;
    The West Australian, 22 July 2003

Rose Rebecca; *Ban junk food ads: expert*; The West Australian, 11 September 2002

Stanton Dr Rosemary; *Chewing the Fat*; Australian Good Taste Magazine; September 2003

Miscellaneous sources

Butylated Hydroxyanisole(BHA) CAS No. 25013-16-5; *Reasonably Anticipated to be a Carcinogen*; Ninth Report on Carcinogens.

Dingle Peter; *2600 Food Additives Course Notes*; July 2003

J Breaky; Review Article - *The role of diet and behaviour in childhood;* Journal of Paediatrics and Child Health 1997;33 (3):190-4

Lau K and others; *Synergistic Interactions Between Commonly Used Food Additives in a Developmental Neurotoxicity Test;* Toxicol Sci 2005: Dec 13

Hermanussen and others; *Obesity, voracity and short stature: the impact of glutamate on the regulation of appetite*; European Journal of Clinical Nutrition, 2005

Bateman B and others; *The effects of a double blind, placebo controlled artificial food colourings and benzoate preservatives challenge on hyperactivity in a general population sample of pre school children*; Archives of Diseases in Childhood 2004; 899: 506 -511

McCann D and others; *Food additives and hyperactive behaviour in 3-year-old and 8/9-year-old children in the community: a randomised, double-blinded, placebo controlled trial*; The Lancet Vol 370, Issue 9598, 3 November 2007, Pages 1560 – 1567

Piper PW; *Yeast superoxide dismutase mutants reveal a pro-oxidant action of weak organic acid food preservatives;* Free Radic Biol Med. 1999 Dec;27(11-12):1219-27. PMID: 10641714

————————————
————————————
————————————
————————————

Chief Executive Officer
Food Standards Australia New Zealand
PO Box 7186
CANBERRA ACT 2610

Dear Sir / Madam,

RE: Full disclosure of ingredients

I am writing to you as a concerned consumer who has recently become aware of serious shortcomings in our food-labelling code administered by your agency. My understanding is that, despite the recent changes to the labelling requirements in this country, there still exists a 5% loophole that enables manufacturers to not disclose fully the ingredients in their products. The current legislation allows for manufacturers not to declare components of ingredients that make up less than 5% of a product or which are determined by the manufacturer as having no technological function.

As a result of this loophole, there are many products on the market that contain food additives that are, quite legally, not declared on the label. Consumers are consequently denied the right to be fully informed about what is in the food we eat. For whatever reasons, many consumers wish to avoid certain substances, and the current legislation doesn't support the consumers' right to full information and choice. Rather, it appears biased in favour of manufacturers.

As the charter of FSANZ is to protect the health and safety of people, I believe that your agency has a clear responsibility to ensure that full-disclosure in labelling is introduced without delay.

Consumers have a right to know what is in the food we purchase, regardless of whether or not additives are deemed safe. It is the responsibility of FSANZ to ensure that the labelling legislation in this country is amended to reflect this change and to require that manufacturers declare all components of their products, no matter how small or what function they are deemed to perform.

Thank you for your consideration of this issue. I look forward to hearing from you regarding the timing for such changes to be implemented by your agency.

Yours sincerely,

....

Some comments from our readers

Since Additive Alert was published in September 2004, we have been inundated with confirmation from all over the country that food additives are playing havoc with the health and well being of Australians, both young and old. Additive Alert does not make any specific health claims, nor do we promise a miracle cure for any health or behaviour problems. However, the anecdotal evidence we receive from everyday real people is undeniably strong. Food additives and diet can play a huge role in alleviating problems for many people.

Here is a small sample of what people have to say about the way food additives effect them and how Additive Alert has helped them. I hope this book will help you too.

****

"I bought your book because my nearly two year old (girl) was such a terrible night time sleeper that I no longer knew what to do with her. So out went the additives and preservatives, along came my bookmark when I went shopping and we began making all our own treats, cakes and biscuits. What a difference it made!!!. My 3 1/2 year old (girl) does not seem to have any of the same issues with much of the food although I did notice the change in their aggressive behaviour within days. Thank you so much."

****

"As a mother of three I have tried to maintain what I thought was a healthy diet for my kids since they were born, insisting on fresh fruit and vegetables and little to no junk food. However, a friend recently bought your book and I was shocked to say the least at how little I really knew, and I was outraged at the fact that FSANZ is basically using our children as guinea pigs. I am sending this email to say THANKYOU for all the hard work and thank you for making me aware of what they put in our food."

****

"My life has been totally transformed since cutting out foods which I thought would be ok even though I knew they would not be of any nutritional value. Its a big statement to say that "I have got my life back" but that is what has happened since I avoided foods containing the worst additives. It is nearly criminal what is being given to us in the name of food. Please put me on your data base."